This book is due for return on or before the last date shown below

D1336408

Burn Care and Treatment

Marc G. Jeschke • Lars-Peter Kamolz
Shahriar Shahrokhi
Editors

Burn Care and Treatment

A Practical Guide

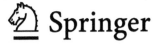 Springer

Editors

Marc G. Jeschke, M.D., Ph.D., FACS,
FCCM, FRCS(C)
Division of Plastic Surgery
Department of Surgery and Immunology
Ross Tilley Burn Centre
Sunnybrook Health Sciences Centre
Sunnybrook Research Institute
University of Toronto
Toronto
ON
Canada

Shahriar Shahrokhi, M.D., FRCSC
Division of Plastic and Reconstructive Surgery
Ross Tilley Burn Centre
Sunnybrook Health Sciences Centre
Toronto
ON
Canada

Lars-Peter Kamolz, M.D., FACS, FCCM,
FRCS(C)
Department of Surgery
Medical University of Graz
Graz
Austria

ISBN 978-3-7091-1132-1   ISBN 978-3-7091-1133-8   (eBook)
DOI 10.1007/978-3-7091-1133-8
Springer Wien Heidelberg New York Dordrecht London

Library of Congress Control Number: 2013933290

Contents

Initial Assessment, Resuscitation, Wound Evaluation and Early Care

Shahriar Shahrokhi

1.1 Initial Assessment and Emergency Treatment

The initial assessment and management of a burn patient begins with prehospital care. There is a great need for efficient and accurate assessment, transportation, and emergency care for these patients in order to improve their overall outcome. Once the initial evaluation has been completed, the transportation to the appropriate care facility is of outmost importance. At this juncture, it is imperative that the patient is transported to facility with the capacity to provide care for the thermally injured patient; however, at times patients would need to be transported to the nearest care facility for stabilization (i.e., airway control, establishment of IV access).

Once in the emergency room, the assessment as with any trauma patient is composed of primary and secondary surveys (Box 1.1). As part of the primary survey, the establishment of a secure airway is paramount. An expert in airway management should accomplish this as these patients can rapidly deteriorate from airway edema.

Box 1.1. Primary and Secondary Survey
Primary survey:
- Airway:
  - Preferably #8 ETT placed orally
  - Always be prepared for possible surgical airway
- Breathing:
  - Ensure proper placement of ETT by auscultation/x-ray
  - Bronchoscopic assessment for inhalation injury

S. Shahrokhi, M.D., FRCSC
Division of Plastic and Reconstructive Surgery,
Ross Tilley Burn Centre, Sunnybrook Health Sciences Centre,
2075 Bayview Ave, Suite D716, Toronto, ON M4N 3M5, Canada
e-mail: shar.shahrokhi@sunnybrook.ca

M.G. Jeschke et al. (eds.), *Burn Care and Treatment*,
DOI 10.1007/978-3-7091-1133-8_1, © Springer-Verlag Wien 2013

- Circulation:
  - Establish adequate IV access (large bore IV placed peripherally in non-burnt tissue if possible, central access would be required but can wait)
  - Begin resuscitation based on the Parkland formula

Secondary survey:
- Complete head to toe assessment of patient
- Obtain information about the patient's past medical history, mediations, allergies, tetanus status
- Determine the circumstances/mechanism of injury
  - Entrapment in closed space
  - Loss of consciousness
  - Time since injury
  - Flame, scald, grease, chemical, electrical
- Examination should include a thorough neurological assessment
- All extremities should be examined to determine possible neurovascular compromise (i.e., possible compartment syndrome) and need for escharotomies
- Burn size and depth should be determined at the end of the survey

Table 1.1 ABA criteria for transfer to a burn unit[a]

1. Partial-thickness burns greater than 10 % total body surface area (TBSA)
2. Burns that involve the face, hands, feet, genitalia, perineum, or major joints
3. Third-degree burns in any age group
4. Electrical burns, including lightning injury
5. Chemical burns
6. Inhalation injury
7. Burn injury in patients with preexisting medical disorders that could complicate management, prolong recovery, or affect mortality
8. Any patient with burns and concomitant trauma (such as fractures) in which the burn injury poses the greatest risk of morbidity or mortality. In such cases, if the trauma poses the greater immediate risk, the patient may be initially stabilized in a trauma center before being transferred to a burn unit. Physician judgment will be necessary in such situations and should be in concert with the regional medical control plan and triage protocols
9. Burned children in hospitals without qualified personnel or equipment for the care of children
10. Burn injury in patients who will require special social, emotional, or rehabilitative intervention

[a]From Ref. [1]

Once this initial assessment is complete, the disposition of the patient will be determined by the ABA criteria for burn unit referral [1] (Table 1.1).

In determining the %TBSA (% total body surface area) burn, the rule of 9 s can be used; however, it is not as accurate as the Lund and Browder chart (Fig. 1.1) which further subdivides the body for a more accurate calculation. First-degree burns are not included.

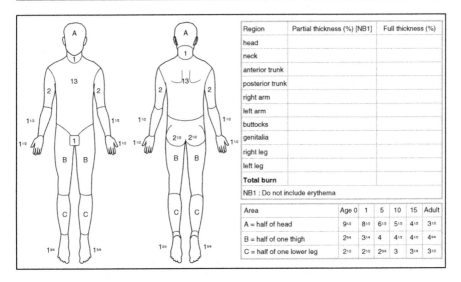

Region	Partial thickness (%) [NB1]	Full thickness (%)
head		
neck		
anterior trunk		
posterior trunk		
right arm		
left arm		
buttocks		
genitalia		
right leg		
left leg		
Total burn		
NB1 : Do not include erythema		

Area	Age 0	1	5	10	15	Adult
A = half of head	9½	8½	6½	5½	4½	3½
B = half of one thigh	2¾	3¼	4	4½	4½	4¾
C = half of one lower leg	2½	2½	2¾	3	3¼	3½

Fig. 1.1 Lund and Browder chart for calculating %TBSA burn

Table 1.2 Typical clinical appearance of burn depth

First-degree burns	Involves only the epidermis and never blisters
	Appears as a "sunburn"
	Is not included in the %TBSA calculation
Second-degree burns (dermal burns)	Superficial
	Pink, homogeneous, normal cap refill, painful, moist, intact hair follicles
	Deep
	Mottled or white, delayed or absent cap refill, dry, decreased sensation or insensate, non-intact hair follicles
Third-degree burns	Dry, white or charred, leathery, insensate

Assessment of burn depth can be precarious even for experts in the field. There are some basics principles, which can help in evaluating the burn depth (Table 1.2). Always be aware that burns are dynamic and burn depth can progress or convert to being deeper. Therefore, reassessment is important in establishing burn depth.

Given that even burn experts are only 64–76 % [2] accurate in determining burn depth, there has been an increased desire to have more objective method of determining burn depth, and therefore, technologies have been and continue to be developed and utilized in this field. These are summarized in the following Table 1.3 [3]:

Once the initial assessment and stabilization are complete, the physician needs to determine the patient's disposition. Those that can be treated as outpatient (do not

Table 1.3 Techniques used for assessment of burn depth[a]

Technique	Advantages	Disadvantages
Radioactive isotopes	Radioactive phosphorus (^{32}P) taken up by the skin	Invasive, too cumbersome, poorly reproducible
Nonfluorescent dyes	Differentiate necrotic from living tissue on the surface	No determination of depth of necrosis; many dyes not approved for clinical use
Fluorescent dyes	Approved for clinical use	Invasive; marks necrosis at a fixed distance in millimeters, not accounting for thickness of the skin; large variability
Thermography	Noninvasive, fast assessment	Many false positives and false negatives based on evaporative cooling and presence of blisters; each center needs to validate its own values
Photometry	Portable, noninvasive, fast assessment, validated against senior burn surgeons, and color palette was developed	Single-institution experience; expensive?
Liquid crystal film	Inexpensive	Contact with tissue required, unreliable readings
Nuclear magnetic resonance	Water content in tissue differentiates partial from full-thickness wounds	In vitro assessment only, expensive, time-consuming
Nuclear imaging	^{99}mTc shows areas of deeper injury	Expensive, very time-consuming, not readily available, and invasive
Pulse-echo ultrasound	Noninvasive, easily available	Underestimates depth of injury, operator-dependent, and requires contact with tissue
Doppler ultrasound	Noncontact technology available, provides morphologic and flow information	Operator-dependent, not as reliable as laser Doppler
Laser Doppler imaging	Noninvasive and noncontact technology, fast assessment, large body of experience in multiple centers, and very accurate prediction in small wounds in stable patients	Readings affected by temperature, distance from wound, wound humidity, angle of recordings, extent of tissue edema, and presence of shock; different versions of the technology available make extrapolation of results difficult

[a]From Jaskille et al. [3]

meet burn unit referral criteria) will need their wounds treated appropriately. There are many choices for outpatient wound therapy, and the choice will be mostly dependent on the availability of products and physician preference/knowledge/comfort with application. Table 1.5 summarizes some of the available products.

The thermally injured patients who are transferred to burn units for treatment will be discussed in the next section on fluid resuscitation and early management.

1.2   Fluid Resuscitation and Early Management

1.2.1   Fluid Resuscitation

As mentioned previously, patients with <10 % TBSA burn do not require fluid resuscitation. However, burn encompassing >15 % TBSA will require fluid resuscitation. Several formulas have been proposed for the resuscitation of the burn patient, all requiring crystalloid infusion with or without the addition of colloids. However, the mainstay of fluid resuscitation remains the Parkland formula:

$$4\ ml \times \%TBSA \times weight\ (kg) = 24\ h\ fluid\ requirement, \text{ with half given over the}$$
$$\text{first 8 h and the remainder over the following 16h}$$

While the Parkland formula provides with the total amount for 24 h and starting level for initiation of resuscitation, it is not an absolute. The fluid resuscitation should be guided by physiological parameters and laboratory findings to prevent under/over-resuscitation. The goals of resuscitation should be restoration of intravascular volume, maintenance of organ perfusion and function, while preventing burn wound conversion.

In resuscitating a thermally injured patient, one must be cognizant of the three components of burn shock: cardiogenic shock, distributive shock, and hypovolemic shock. Each has a fundamental role in the pathophysiology of the burn patient and cannot be treated in a similar fashion. The myocardial depressant effects of inflammatory mediators post-burn injury has been well documented [4–8]. This typically last up to 36 h following which the patients' cardiac function typically becomes hyper-dynamic.

Therefore, during the initial phase of burn resuscitation, the physician not only has to restore the patients' intravascular volume but also might need to consider inotropic agents to aid the myocardial dysfunction.

1.2.2   Endpoint of Burn Resuscitation

Traditionally the endpoints of resuscitation of a thermally injured patient have been determined via physiological parameters; however, the use of global end-organ functions such as urinary output, heart rate, and blood pressure is inadequate in determining the adequacy of resuscitation [9]. The addition of measurements of base deficit and lactate has become commonplace as markers of adequate resuscitation; however, it is difficult to ascertain their importance as markers of burn resuscitation as there are multiple episodes of ischemia and reperfusion injury with fluctuation in serum lactate and base deficit level [10]. In some studies, it appears that elevated lactate and base deficit levels on admission do correlate with overall organ dysfunction and mortality; however, there is no absolute number or threshold, which determines non-survivability [11–14]. Moreover, further studies have concluded that elevated lactate level is an independent risk factor for mortality [15–17].

Since at this juncture, there is no ideal method for determining the endpoints of resuscitation, some researchers have begun to adopt new techniques. Light et al.

demonstrated the use of tissue pCO_2 monitoring to better correlate with tissue perfusion; however, its use is not commonplace as yet [10].

Clinical assessment is outdated; the use of resuscitation markers (BD, and lactate) is flawed; however, there are some which correlate well with overall risk of organ dysfunction and mortality. Newer techniques are under examination but have not gained wide acceptance for use. In conclusion, until a widely accepted method has been validated, care must be taken to incorporate as many tools as possible to determine adequate resuscitation.

1.2.3 Fluid Over-resuscitation and Fluid Creep

The mainstay of fluid resuscitation remains crystalloid solutions (mainly Ringer's lactate). However, consideration should be given to colloids if the resuscitation volumes are far exceeding those set out by the Parkland calculation as not to endure the consequences of fluid creep [18] such as:

- Abdominal compartment syndrome (ACS) [19–23]
- Extremity compartment syndrome [24]
- Respiratory failure and prolonged intubation [24]
- Pulmonary edema and pleural effusions [24]
- Orbital compartment syndrome [25]

One of the more dire consequences of fluid creep is ACS, with resultant mortality of 70–100 % [19, 22, 26–29]. Some of the strategies that can be utilized to decrease risk of ACS or prevent IAH (intra-abdominal hypertension) progressing to ACS in a burn patient are:

- Vigilant monitoring of fluid resuscitation – decrease fluid volumes as quickly as possible
- Monitor intra-abdominal pressures in all patients with >30 % TBSA burn
- Perform escharotomies on full-thickness torso burns and proceed to a "checkerboard pattern" if inadequate
- Consider aggressive diuresis if evidence of over-resuscitation
- Consider neuromuscular blockade to alleviate abdominal muscle tone

Should all the above strategies fail in lowering the intra-abdominal pressure, the definitive solution is a decompressive laparotomy with aforementioned mortality of up to 100 % [19, 22, 26–29]. As a result, many have looked at other modes of resuscitation beyond the use of crystalloid solutions.

1.2.4 Role of Colloids, Hypertonic Saline, and Antioxidants in Resuscitation

1.2.4.1 Colloids

As mentioned previously, the initial resuscitation is accomplished with mainly crystalloids. This is mainly as the consequence of burn pathophysiology, whereby there is a significant increase in the permeability of capillaries post-thermal injury with resultant movement shift of fluid into the interstitial space [30–35]. This increase permeability appears to resolve in 8–12 h post-injury. Typically, colloids are not recommended in the initial 12 h phase of resuscitation (however, there is no clear evidence as to the exact timing for initiation of colloids).

The colloid of choice is albumin (5 % concentration), given as an infusion to decrease the crystalloid requirements. There is some evidence that use of colloids in the resuscitation of the thermally injured patient does normalize the I/O ratios; however, the effect on morbidity and mortality is unknown at this time [36, 37]. In critical care literature, which typically excludes the burn patients, the studies have shown that the use of colloids is safe with no overall benefit to the patient [38], and the Cochrane review in 2011 concluded that "there is no evidence that albumin reduces mortality in patients with hypovolemia, burns or hypoproteinemia. For patients with burns or hypoproteinemia, there is a suggestion that albumin administration may increase mortality" [39]. So despite the extensive of use of albumin in burn resuscitation, there is paucity of evidence for its use, and the overall benefit remains controversial.

1.2.4.2 Hypertonic Saline
The role of hypertonic saline in burn resuscitation has been studied greatly with variable results. In recent years, there has been a shift in thinking in the use of hypertonic saline. Rather than using hypertonic saline as the sole resuscitative fluid with goals of reducing fluid requirements, it has been studied in the context of decreasing the inflammatory response and bacterial translocation and therefore infectious complications [40–42].

1.2.4.3 Antioxidants: High-Dose Vitamin C
It is well documented that following thermal injury, there is an increased in capillary permeability leading to edema. The initial studies conducted by Tanaka et al. and Matsuda et al. indicated the lower water content of burn wounds with high-dose vitamin C infusion, with decreased overall resuscitation fluid requirements [43–46]. More recently, studies have demonstrated that resuscitation with high-dose vitamin C reduces the endothelial damage post-thermal injury [47, 48], with decrease in overall fluid volumes administered with no increase in morbidity or mortality [48, 49].

In summary, the resuscitation of the burn patient is complex and requires use of all tools available. It can no longer be the domain of crystalloid resuscitation without consideration for colloids, hypertonic saline, and high-dose vitamin C along with other antioxidants. All aspects of burn shock requires treatment (not just the hypovolemic component), which might require the early use of vasopressors and inotropes. Finally, the end goals of resuscitation need to be better monitored to assess the effectiveness of the resuscitation and ensure improved patient outcomes.

1.3   Evaluation and Early Management of Burn Wound

1.3.1   Evaluation of Burn Depth

The evaluation of the burn wound is of utmost importance, and expert clinicians have been known to be incorrect in their assessment up to 30 % of the time.

Table 1.4 Clinical appearance of dermal and full-thickness burns

Clinical appearance	Superficial dermal	Deep dermal	Full thickness
Presence of blisters	Yes	Yes	No
Dermal depth	Papillary	Reticular	Entire depth
Color of exposed dermis	Pink	Mottled/white	White/charred/leathery
Capillary refill	Yes	Delayed/none	None
Time to heal	<21 days	>21 days	>21 days
Moisture	Moist	Dry	Dry
Pain	Very painful	Minimal to none	Insensate
Dermal appendages	Intact	Not intact	Not intact

As previously indicated, multiple modalities have been examined to determine their efficacy and possible role in the determination of the burn depth (Table 1.3), but none has replaced the clinical examination as gold standard.

In general, first-degree burns are of minimal concern. They only involve the epidermis with erythema and no blisters and do not require medical attention. Second-degree burns (dermal burns) and beyond are those that will require medical attention. Dermal burns are divided into superficial and deep. Their clinical characteristics are summarized in Table 1.4.

The depth of the burn determines not only the requirement for admission but also the management – operative versus conservative. The ideal treatment for all burns, which will not heal between 14 and 21 days, is to have operative excision and skin grafting. All others can be treated conservatively. The conservative management of burns includes appropriate wound care and therapy for maintenance of range of motion and overall function.

1.3.2 Choice of Topical Dressings

There are various topical agents that are available for management of burns. Typically, the topical management of deep burns requires an antimicrobial agent to minimize bacterial colonization and hence infection. For superficial burns, the goal of the topical agent is to reduce environmental factors causing pain and provide the appropriate environment for wound healing. Table 1.5 summarizes some of the agents available for topical treatment of burns, and the choice of agent is dependent on their availability and the comfort and knowledge of the caregivers.

The choice of burn dressing needs to take into account the following factors:
- Eliminate the environmental factors causing pain
- Act as barrier to environmental flora
- Reduce evaporative losses
- Absorb and contain drainage
- Provide splinting to maintain position of function
The goals of topical antimicrobial therapy for deep dermal and full-thickness burns:
- To delay/minimize wound colonization
- Have the ability to penetrate eschar

Table 1.5 Topical therapy for treatment of cutaneous burns

Agent	Description
Bacitracin/polymyxin B	Ointment for superficial burns
Mupirocin	2 % Ointment for superficial burns
	Activity against MRSA
Biobrane	Artificial skin substitute bilayer – silicone film with a nylon fabric outer layer and a tri-filament thread with collagen bound inner layer
	For treatment of superficial dermal burns, Biobrane can be left intact until wound fully healed
	Reduces pain and evaporative losses
Aquacel *Ag*	Methylcellulose dressing with ionic silver for superficial dermal burns
	Can be left intact until wound fully healed
	Wound base needs to be clean for dressing adherence
Silver sulfadiazine	1 % cream for deep dermal and full-thickness burns
	Has broad spectrum of activity
	Intermediate eschar penetration
Mafenide acetate	Available as 11 % water-soluble cream or 5 % solution for deep dermal and full-thickness burns
	Has broad spectrum of activity, however, minimal activity against staphylococcus species
	Excellent eschar penetration
Acticoat	Sheet of thin, flexible rayon/polyester bonded with silver crystal-embedded polyethylene mesh
	Can be left on the wound for 3–7 days
	Has broad-spectrum activity

- Have activity against common pathogens
  - *S. aureus, Proteus, Klebsiella, E. coli, Pseudomonas*
- Should not retard wound healing
- Have low toxicity (minimal systemic absorption)

1.3.3 Escharotomy

In evaluation of wounds, consideration also needs to be given for possible need for escharotomy. All deep circumferential burns to the extremity have the potential to cause neurovascular compromise and therefore benefit from escharotomies. The typical clinical signs of impaired perfusion in the burned extremity/hand include cool temperature, decreased or absent capillary refill, tense compartments, with the hand held in the claw position, and absence of pulses is a late sign [52]. On occasion, non-circumferential deep burns or circumferential partial-thickness burns might require a prophylactic escharotomy as the patient might require large resuscitation volumes due to overall injury or the inability to perform serial reassessments [52].

Escharotomies of the extremities are performed along the medial and lateral lines, with the extremity held in the anatomic position. For the hand, the escharotomy is performed along the second and fourth metacarpals, and for the fingers, care is taken to prevent any neurovascular damage; therefore, escharotomies are typically not performed along the ulnar aspect of the thumb or the radial aspect of the index finger [50–52].

1.3.4 Operative Management

Once the thermally injured patient has been admitted, resuscitated, all wounds assessed, and managed appropriately with escharotomy and dressing, the surgeons needs to determine the most efficient course of action in regard to excision of burn and coverage. This needs to be undertaken as soon as patient is resuscitated usually within 24–48 h post-injury.

References

1. Committee on Trauma, American College of Surgeons (2006) Guidelines for the operation of burn centers, resources for optimal care of the injured patient. American College of Surgeons, Chicago, pp 79–86
2. Heimbach DM, Afromowitz MA, Engrav LH, Marvin JA, Perry B (1984) Burn depth estimation – man or machine. J Trauma 24:373–378
3. Jaskille AD, Ramella-Roman JC, Shupp JW, Jordan MH, Jeng JC (2010) Critical review of burn depth assessment techniques: part II. Review of laser Doppler technology. J Burn Care Res 31:151–157
4. Hilton JG, Marullo DS (1986) Effects of thermal trauma on cardiac force of contraction. Burns Incl Therm Inj 12:167–171
5. Papp A, Uusaro A, Parvianen I et al (2003) Myocardial function and hemodynamics in extensive burn trauma: evaluation by clinical signs, invasive monitoring, echocardiography, and cytokine concentrations. A prospective clinical study. Acta Anesthesiol Scand 47: 1257–1263
6. Adams HR, Baxter CR, Izenberg SD (1984) Decreased contractility and compliance of the left ventricle as complications of thermal trauma. Am Heart J 108:1477–1487
7. Horton J, Maass D, White DJ et al (2006) Effect of aspiration pneumonia: induced sepsis on post burn cardiac inflammation and function in mice. Surg Infect (Larchmt) 7:123–135
8. Huang YS, Yang ZC, Yan BG et al (1999) Pathogenesis of early cardiac myocyte damage after severe burns. J Trauma 46:428–432
9. Dries DJ, Waxman K (1991) Adequate resuscitation for burn patients may not be measured by urine output and vital signs. Crit Care Med 19:327–329
10. Light TD, Jeng JC, Jain AK, Jablonski KA, Kim DE, Phillips TM, Rizzo AG, Jordan MH (2004) Real-time metabolic monitors, ischemia-reperfusion, titration endpoints, and ultraprecise burn resuscitation. J Burn Care Rehabil 25:33–44

11. Jeng JC, Lee K, Jablonski K et al (1997) Serum lactate and base deficit suggest inadequate resuscitation of patients with burn injuries: application of a point-of-care laboratory instrument. J Burn Care Rehabil 18:402–405
12. Choi J, Cooper A, Gomez M et al (2000) The relevance of base deficits after burn injuries. J Burn Care Rehabil 21:499–505
13. Cartotto R, Choi J, Gomez M, Cooper A (2003) A prospective study on the implications of a base deficit during fluid resuscitation. J Burn Care Rehabil 24:75–84
14. Kaups KL, Davis JW, Dominic WJ (1998) Base deficit as an indicator of resuscitation needs in patients with burn injuries. J Burn Care Rehabil 19:346–348
15. Jeng JC, Jablonski K, Bridgeman A, Jordan MH (2002) Serum lactate, not base deficit, rapidly predicts survival after major burns. Burns 28:161–166
16. Kamolz L-P, Andel H, Schramm W et al (2005) Lactate: early predictor of morbidity and mortality in patients with severe burns. Burns 31:986–990
17. Cochran A, Edelman S, Saffle JR, Stephen E, Morris SE (2007) The relationship of serum lactate and base deficit in burn patients to mortality. J Burn Care Res 28:231–240
18. Saffle JR (2007) The phenomenon of fluid creep in acute burn resuscitation. J Burn Care Res 28:382–395
19. Hobson KG, Young KM, Ciraulo A et al (2002) Release of abdominal compartment syndrome improves survival in patients with burn injury. J Trauma 53:1129–1134
20. Greenhalgh DG, Warden GD (1994) The importance of intra-abdominal pressure measurements in burned children. J Trauma 36:685–690
21. Ivy ME, Possenti PP, Kepros J et al (1999) Abdominal compartment syndrome in patients with burns. J Burn Care Rehabil 20:351–353
22. Oda J, Ueyama M, Yamashita K et al (2005) Effects of escharotomy as abdominal decompression on cardiopulmonary function and visceral perfusion in abdominal compartment syndrome with burn patients. J Trauma 59:369–374
23. Jensen AR, Hughes WB, Grewal H (2006) Secondary abdominal compartment syndrome in children with burns and trauma: a potentially lethal combination. J Burn Care Res 27:242–246
24. Zak AL, Harrington DL, Barillo DJ et al (1999) Acute respiratory failure that complicates the resuscitation of pediatric patients with scald injuries. J Burn Care Rehabil 20:391–399
25. Sullivan SR, Ahmadi AJ, Singh CN et al (2006) Elevated orbital pressure: another untoward effect of massive resuscitation after burn injury. J Trauma 60:72–76
26. Malbrain ML, Cheatham ML, Kirkpatrick A et al (2006) Results from the international conference of experts on intra-abdominal hypertension and abdominal compartment syndrome 1. Definitions. Intensive Care Med 32:1722–1732
27. Ivy ME, Atweh NA, Palmer J et al (2000) Intra-abdominal hypertension and abdominal compartment syndrome in burn patients. J Trauma 49:387–391
28. Latenser BA, Kowal-Vern A, Kimball D et al (2002) A pilot study comparing percutaneous decompression with decompressive laparotomy for acute abdominal compartment syndrome. J Burn Care Rehabil 23:190–195
29. Hershberger RC, Hunt JL, Arnoldo BD et al (2007) Abdominal compartment syndrome in the severely burned patient. J Burn Care Res 28:708–714
30. Demling RH (2005) The burn edema process: current concepts. J Burn Care Res 26:207–227
31. Carvajal HF, Linares HA, Brouhard BH (1979) Relationship of burn size to vascular permeability changes in rats. Surg Gynecol Obstet 149:193–202
32. Demling RH, Kramer GC, Harms B (1984) Role of thermal injury induced hypoproteinemia on fluid flux and protein permeability in burned and nonburned tissue. Surgery 95:136–144
33. Lund T, Onarkeim H, Reed R (1992) Pathogenesis of edema formation in burn injuries. World J Surg 16:2–9
34. Cope O, Moore F (1944) A study of capillary permeability in experimental burns and burn shock using radioactive dyes in blood and lymph. J Clin Invest 23:241–249
35. Bert J, Bowen B, Reed R et al (1991) Microvascular exchange during burn injury: fluid resuscitation model. Circ Shock 37:285–297

36. Lawrence A, Faraklas I, Watkins H, Allen A, Cochran A, Morris S, Saffle J (2010) Colloid administration normalizes resuscitation ratio and ameliorates "fluid creep". J Burn Care Res 31:40–47

37. Faraklas I, Lam U, Cochran A, Stoddard G, Jeffrey Saffle J (2011) Colloid normalizes resuscitation ratio in pediatric burns. J Burn Care Res 32:91–97

38. The SAFE Study Investigators (2004) A comparison of albumin and saline for fluid resuscitation in the intensive care unit. N Engl J Med 350:2247–2256

39. Roberts I, Blackhall K, Alderson P, Bunn F, Schierhout G. Human albumin solution for resuscitation and volume expansion in critically ill patients. Cochrane Database of Systematic Reviews 2011, Issue 11. Art. No.: CD001208. DOI:10.1002/14651858.CD001208.pub4

40. Chen LW, Hwang B, Wang JS, Chen JS, Hsu CM (2004) Hypertonic saline-enhanced postburn gut barrier failure is reversed by inducible nitric oxide synthase inhibition. Crit Care Med 32(12):2476–2484

41. Chen LW, Huang HL, Lee IT, Hsu CM, Lu PJ (2006) Hypertonic saline enhances host defense to bacterial challenge by augmenting toll-like receptors. Crit Care Med 34(6):1758–1768

42. Chen LW, Su MT, Chen PH, Liu WC, Hsu CM (2011) Hypertonic saline enhances host defense and reduces apoptosis in burn mice by increasing toll-like receptors. Shock 35(1):59–66

43. Matsuda T, Tanaka H, Williams S, Hanumadass M, Abcarian H, Reyes H (1991) Reduced fluid volume requirement for resuscitation of third-degree burns with high-dose vitamin C. J Burn Care Rehabil 12(6):525–532

44. Matsuda T, Tanaka H, Shimazaki S, Matsuda H, Abcarian H, Reyes H, Hanumadass M (1992) High-dose vitamin C therapy for extensive deep dermal burns. Burns 18(2):127–131

45. Tanaka H, Matsuda H, Shimazaki S, Hanumadass M, Matsuda T (1997) Reduced resuscitation fluid volume for second-degree burns with delayed initiation of ascorbic acid therapy. Arch Surg 132(2):158–161

46. Sakurai M, Tanaka H, Matsuda T, Goya T, Shimazaki S, Matsuda H (1997) Reduced resuscitation fluid volume for second-degree experimental burns with delayed initiation of vitamin C therapy (beginning 6 h after injury). J Surg Res 73(1):24–27

47. Dubick MA, Williams C, Elgjo GI, Kramer GC (2005) High-dose vitamin C infusion reduces fluid requirements in the resuscitation of burn-injured sheep. Shock 24(2):139–144

48. Kremer T, Harenberg P, Hernekamp F, Riedel K, Gebhardt MM, Germann G, Heitmann C, Walther A (2010) High-dose vitamin C treatment reduces capillary leakage after burn plasma transfer in rats. J Burn Care Res 31(3):470–479

49. Kahn SA, Beers RJ, Lentz CW (2011) Resuscitation after severe burn injury using high-dose ascorbic acid: a retrospective review. J Burn Care Res 32(1):110–117

50. Sheridan RL, Hurley J, Smith MA et al (1995) The acutely burned hand: management and outcomes based on a ten-year experience with 1047 acute hand burns. J Trauma 38:406–411

51. Smith MA, Munster AM, Spence RJ (1998) Burns of the hand and upper limb – a review. Burns 24:493–505

52. Cartotto R (2005) The burned hand: optimizing long-term outcomes with a standardized approach to acute and subacute care. Clin Plast Surg 32:515–527

Pathophysiology of Burn Injury

2

Marc G. Jeschke

2.1 Introduction

Advances in therapy strategies, due to improved understanding of resuscitation, enhanced wound coverage, better support of hypermetabolic response to injury, more appropriate infection control, and improved treatment of inhalation injury, based on better understanding of the pathophysiologic responses to burn injury have further improved the clinical outcome of this unique patient population over the past years [1]. This chapter describes the present understanding of the pathophysiology of a burn injury including both the local and systemic responses, focusing on the many facets of organ and systemic effects directly resulting from hypovolemia and circulating mediators following burn trauma.

2.2 Local Changes

2.2.1 Temperature and Time Effect

Local changes appear in the tissue when the amount of absorbed heat exceeds the body system's compensatory mechanisms. On a molecular level, protein degradation begins at a temperature of 40 °C. This degradation leads to alterations in cell homeostasis. This

M.G. Jeschke, MD, PhD, FACS, FCCM, FRCS(C)
Division of Plastic Surgery, Department of Surgery and Immunology,
Ross Tilley Burn Centre, Sunnybrook Health Sciences Centre,
Sunnybrook Research Institute, University of Toronto,
Rm D704, Bayview Ave. 2075, M4N 3M5, Toronto, ON, Canada
e-mail: marc.jeschke@sunnybrook.ca

M.G. Jeschke et al. (eds.), *Burn Care and Treatment*,
DOI 10.1007/978-3-7091-1133-8_2, © Springer-Verlag Wien 2013

is reversible if the temperature is lowered. Starting at 45 °C, proteins are permanently denatured. This is reflected by local tissue necrosis. The speed with which permanent tissue damage can appear is dependent on the time of exposure and temperature.

45–51 °C	Within minutes
51 and 70 °C	Within seconds
Above 70 °C	Less than a second

The depth and severity of the burn are also determined by the ability of the contact material to transfer heat, a factor referred to as the specific heat. This is especially important in scald and contact burns. The knowledge about the material type allows for a more accurate estimate of tissue damage.

Definition: Burn depth is determined by the time of exposure, the temperature at which the burn occurred, and the caloric equivalent of the burn media.

Another determinant of the severity of burn is the location of the burn wound and the age of the burned patient. The thickness of the skin layers increases from the age of 5 up to the age of 50. In elderly patients, the thickness starts to decrease at the age of 65. The epidermis can vary by location from 0.03 up to 0.4 mm. Clinically, the severity of burn injury can be categorized by the differences in the tissue damage and is determined by the depth of the burn.

(a) I degree: superficial burn of the epidermis

First-degree burns are painful, erythematous, and blanch to the touch with an intact epidermal barrier. Examples include sunburn or a minor scald from a kitchen accident. These burns do not result in scarring, and treatment is aimed at comfort with the use of topical soothing salves with or without aloe and oral nonsteroidal anti-inflammatory agents.

(b) IIa degree: burn including epidermis and superficial dermis

(c) IIb degree: burn including epidermis and deep dermis

Second-degree burns are divided into two types: superficial and deep. All second-degree burns have some degree of dermal damage, by definition, and the division is based on the depth of injury into the dermis. Superficial dermal burns are erythematous, painful, blanch to touch, and often blister. Examples include scald injuries from overheated bathtub water and flash flame burns. These wounds spontaneously re-epithelialize from retained epidermal structures in the rete ridges, hair follicles, and sweat glands in 1–2 weeks. After healing, these burns may have some slight skin discoloration over the long term. Deep dermal burns into the reticular dermis appear more pale and mottled, do not blanch to touch, but remain painful to pinprick. These burns heal in 2–5 weeks by reepithelialization from hair follicles and sweat gland keratinocytes, often with severe scarring as a result of the loss of dermis.

(d) III degree: burn including epidermis and dermis and subcuticular layer

Third-degree burns are full thickness through the epidermis and dermis and are characterized by a hard, leathery eschar that is painless and black, white, or cherry red.

No epidermal or dermal appendages remain; thus, these wounds must heal by reepithelialization from the wound edges. Deep dermal and full-thickness burns require excision with skin grafting from the patient to heal the wounds in a timely fashion.

(e) IV degree: all dermal layers including fascia, muscles, and/or bones

Fourth-degree burns involve other organs beneath the skin, such as muscle, bone, and brain.

Currently, burn depth is most accurately assessed by judgment of experienced practitioners. Accurate depth determination is critical to wound healing as wounds that will heal with local treatment are treated differently than those requiring operative intervention. Examination of the entire wound by the physicians ultimately responsible for their management then is the gold standard used to guide further treatment decisions. New technologies, such as the multisensor laser Doppler flowmeter, hold promise for quantitatively determining burn depth.

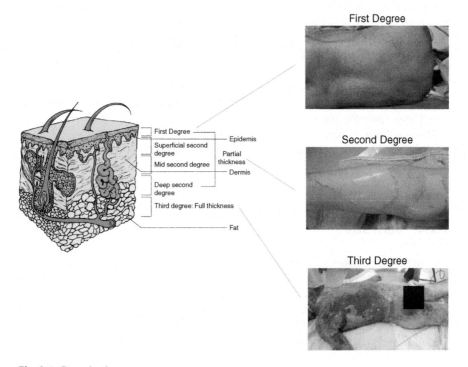

Fig. 2.1 Burn depth

2.2.2 Etiology

The causes include injury from flame (fire), hot liquids (scald), contact with hot or cold objects, chemical exposure, and/or conduction of electricity. The first three induce cellular damage by the transfer of energy, which induces a coagulation necrosis. Chemical burns and electrical burns cause direct injury to cellular membranes in addition to the transfer of heat.

2.2.3 Pathophysiologic Changes

The area of cutaneous or superficial injury has been divided into three zones: zone of coagulation, zone of stasis, and zone of hyperemia. The necrotic area of burn where cells have been disrupted is termed the *zone of coagulation*. This tissue is irreversibly damaged at the time of injury.

The area immediately surrounding the necrotic zone has a moderate degree of insult with decreased tissue perfusion. This is termed the *zone of stasis* and, depending on the wound environment, can either survive or go on to coagulation necrosis. The zone of stasis is associated with vascular damage and vessel leakage [2, 3]. This area is of great importance as this area determines the injury depth of the burned skin. It is important to note that over-resuscitation and increased edema formation can increase the depth of burn, and hence the zone of coagulation and fluids should not only be restricted to avoid pulmonary edema and abdominal compartment syndromes but also to minimize the progressive damage to the burned skin. Other means to attenuate the damage and prevent progression are antioxidants, bradykinin antagonists, and negative wound pressures that improve blood flow and affect the depth of injury [4–6]. Local endothelial interactions with neutrophils mediate some of the local inflammatory responses associated with the zone of stasis. Treatment directed at the control of local inflammation immediately after injury may spare the zone of stasis.

The last area is the *zone of hyperemia,* which is characterized by vasodilation from inflammation surrounding the burn wound. This region contains the clearly viable tissue from which the healing process begins and is generally not at risk for further necrosis.

2.2.4 Burn Size

Determination of burn size estimates the extent of injury. Burn size is generally assessed by the "rule of nines." In adults, each upper extremity and the head and neck are 9 % of the TBSA, the lower extremities and the anterior and posterior trunk are 18 % each, and the perineum and genitalia are assumed to be 1 % of the TBSA. Another method of estimating smaller burns is to equate the area of the open hand (including the palm and the extended fingers) of the patient to be approximately 1 % TBSA and then to transpose that measurement visually onto the wound for a determination of its size. This method is crucial when evaluating burns of mixed distribution. Children have a relatively larger portion of the body surface area in the head and neck, which is compensated for by a relatively smaller surface area in the lower extremities. Infants have 21 % of the TBSA in the head and neck and 13 % in each leg, which incrementally approaches the adult proportions with increasing age. The Berkow formula is used to accurately determine burn size in children.

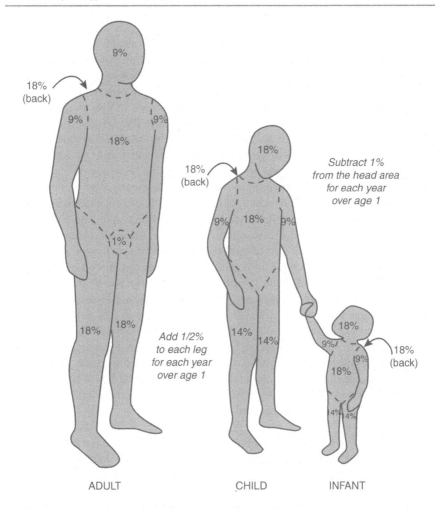

Fig. 2.2 Determination % Body surface area burned. From Handbook-Springer Jeschke eds

2.3   Systemic Changes

2.3.1   Edema Formation

The release of cytokines and other inflammatory mediators at the site of injury has a systemic effect once the burn reaches 20–30 % of total body surface area (TBSA) resulting in severe and unique derangements of cardiovascular function called burn shock. Burn shock is a complex process of circulatory and microcirculatory dysfunction that is not easily or fully repaired by fluid resuscitation. Severe burn injury results in significant hypovolemic shock and substantial tissue trauma, both of which cause the formation and release of many local and systemic mediators [1, 7, 8]. Burn shock results from the interplay of hypovolemia and the release of multiple mediators of inflammation with effects on both the microcirculation as well as the function of the heart, large vessels, and lungs. Subsequently, burn shock continues as a significant pathophysiologic state, even if hypovolemia is corrected. Increases in pulmonary and systemic vascular resistance (SVR) and myocardial depression occur despite adequate preload and volume support [9–12]. Such cardiovascular dysfunctions can further exacerbate the whole-body inflammatory response into a vicious cycle of accelerating organ dysfunction [1, 9–12].

Burn injury causes extravasation of plasma into the burn wound and the surrounding tissues. Extensive burn injuries are hypovolemic in nature and characterized by the hemodynamic changes similar to those that occur after hemorrhage, including decreased plasma volume, cardiac output, urine output, and an increased systemic vascular resistance with resultant reduced peripheral blood flow [1, 9–12]. However, as opposed to a fall in hematocrit with hemorrhagic hypovolemia due to transcapillary refill, an increase in hematocrit and hemoglobin concentration will often appear even with adequate fluid resuscitation. As in the treatment of other forms of hypovolemic shock, the primary initial therapeutic goal is to quickly restore vascular volume and to preserve tissue perfusion in order to minimize tissue ischemia. In extensive burns (>20–30 %TBSA), fluid resuscitation is complicated not only by the severe burn wound edema but also by extravasated and sequestered fluid and protein in non-burned soft tissue. Large volumes of resuscitation solutions are required to maintain vascular volume during the first several hours after an extensive burn. Data suggests that despite fluid resuscitation, normal blood volume is not restored until 24–48 h after large burns.

Edema develops when the rate by which fluid is filtered out of the microvessels exceeds the flow in the lymph vessels draining the same tissue mass. Edema formation often follows a biphasic pattern. An immediate and rapid increase in the water content of burn tissue is seen in the first hour after burn injury [13–15]. A second and more gradual increase in fluid flux of both the burned skin and non-burned soft tissue occurs during the first 12–24 h following burn trauma. The amount of edema formation in burned skin depends on the type and extent of injury and whether fluid resuscitation is provided as well as the type and volume of fluid administered. However, fluid resuscitation elevates blood flow and capillary pressure contributing to further fluid extravasation [14, 15]. Without sustained delivery of fluid into the circulation, edema fluid is somewhat self-limited as plasma volume and capillary pressure decrease. The edema development in thermal injured skin is characterized by the extreme rapid onset of tissue water content, which can double within the first hour after burn [14, 15, 16]. Leape and colleagues found a 70–80 % water content increase in a full-thickness burn wound 30 min after burn injury with 90 % of this change occurring in the first 5 min [16]. There was little increase in burn wound water content after the first hour in the non-resuscitated animals. In resuscitated animals or animals with small wounds, adequate tissue perfusion continues to "feed" the edema for several hours. Demling and others used dichromatic absorptiometry to measure edema development during the first week after an experimental partial-thickness burn injury on one hind limb in sheep [14]. Even though edema was rapid with over 50 % occurring in the first hour, maximum water content did not occur until 12–24 h after burn injury.

2.3.2 Hemodynamic and Cardiac Changes Post-Burn

The cause of reduced cardiac output (CO) during the resuscitative phase of burn injury has been the subject of considerable debate. There is an immediate depression of cardiac output before any detectable reduction in plasma volume [9, 10]. The rapidity of this response suggests a neurogenic response to receptors in the thermally injured skin or increased circulating vasoconstrictor mediators. Soon after injury, a developing hypovolemia and reduced venous return undeniably contribute to the reduced cardiac output. The subsequent persistence of reduced CO after apparently adequate fluid therapy, as evidenced by a reduction in heart rate and restoration of both arterial blood pressure and urinary output, has been attributed to circulating myocardial depressant factor(s), which possibly originates from the burn wound. Demling and colleagues showed a 15 % reduction in CO despite an aggressive volume replacement protocol after a 40 % scald burn in sheep [15]. However, there are also sustained increases in catecholamine secretion and elevated systemic vascular resistance for up to 5 days after burn injury [12, 17]. We recently conducted two clinical studies measuring CO and SVR in severely burned patients and showed that CO fell shortly after injury and then returned toward normal; however, reduced CO did not parallel the blood volume deficit [9, 10]. We concluded that the depression of CO resulted not only from decreased blood volume and venous return but also from an increased SVR. Thus, there are multiple factors that can significantly reduce CO after burn injury. However, resuscitated patients suffering major burn injury can also have supranormal CO from 2–6 days post-injury. This is secondary to the establishment of a hypermetabolic state [9, 10].

Immediately post-burn, patients have low cardiac output characteristic of early shock [18]. However, 3–4 days post-burn, cardiac outputs are 1.5 times greater than that of non-burned, healthy volunteers [9–11]. Heart rates of pediatric burned patients' approach are 1.6 times greater than that of non-burned, healthy volunteers. Post-burn, patients have increased cardiac work [19, 20]. Myocardial oxygen consumption surpasses that of marathon runners and is sustained well into rehabilitative period [19, 21].

Myocardial function can be compromised after burn injury due to overload of the right heart and direct depression of contractility. Increases in the afterload of both the left and right heart result from SVR and PVR elevations. The left ventricle compensates, and CO can be maintained with increased afterload by augmented adrenergic stimulation and increased myocardial oxygen extraction. Burn injury greater than 30 % TBSA can induce intrinsic contractile defects that cannot be corrected by early and adequate fluid resuscitation [22, 23]. Horton also showed more recently that also the left heart can suffer from contractile dysfunction in isolated, coronary perfused, guinea pig hearts harvested 24 h after burn injury [22]. This dysfunction was more pronounced in hearts from aged animals and was not reversed by resuscitation with isotonic fluid. It was largely reversed by treatment with 4 ml/kg of hypertonic saline dextran (HSD), but only if administered during the initial 4–6 h of resuscitation. The authors also effectively ameliorated the cardiac dysfunction of thermal injury with infusions of antioxidants, arginine, and calcium channel blockers [23]. Various other resuscitation and cardiac function studies emphasize the importance of early and adequate fluid therapy and suggest that functional myocardial depression after burn injury maybe alleviated in patients receiving early and adequate volume therapy.

A recent more study delineated the importance of intact cardiac function. The authors compared various burn sizes and the pathophysiologic differences between the burn sizes. They found that the patient with larger burns showed significant worse cardiac function which was the only significant difference in terms of organ function indicating that the heart plays an important role and that cardiac dysfunction is present in large burns and should be accounted for [24].

We therefore suggest to use Dobutamin for impaired cardiac function, beta blocker for tachycardia and catecholamine blockade, and adequate resuscitation and maintenance of appropriate hemoglobin levels.

2.3.3 Hypermetabolic Response Post-Burn

Marked and sustained increases in catecholamine, glucocorticoid, glucagon, and dopamine secretion are thought to initiate the cascade of events leading to the acute hypermetabolic stress response with its ensuing catabolic state [25–34]. The cause of this complex response is not well understood. However, cytokines, endotoxin, reactive oxygen species, nitric oxide, and coagulation as well as complement cascades have also been implicated in regulating this response to burn injury [35]. Once these cascades are initiated, their mediators and by-products appear to stimulate the persistent and increased metabolic rate associated with altered glucose, protein, and lipid metabolism seen after severe burn injury [36]. Several studies have indicated that these metabolic phenomena post-burn occur in a timely manner, suggesting two distinct pattern of metabolic regulation following injury [37].

The first phase occurs within the first 48 h of injury and has classically been called the "ebb phase," [18, 37] characterized by decreases in cardiac output, oxygen consumption, and metabolic rate as well as impaired glucose tolerance associated with its hyperglycemic state. These metabolic variables gradually increase within the first 5 days post-injury to a plateau phase (called the "flow" phase), characteristically associated with hyperdynamic circulation and the above-mentioned hypermetabolic state. Insulin release during this time period was found to be twice that of controls in response to glucose load [38, 39], and plasma glucose levels are markedly elevated, indicating the development of an insulin resistance [40, 41].

Current understanding has been that these metabolic alterations resolve soon after complete wound closure. However, we found in recent studies that sustained hypermetabolic alterations post-burn, indicated by persistent elevations of total urine cortisol levels, serum cytokines, catecholamines, and basal energy requirements, were accompanied by impaired glucose metabolism and insulin sensitivity that persisted for up to 3 years after the initial burn injury [42].

2.3.3.1 Resting Energy Expenditure

For severely burned patients, the resting metabolic rate at thermal neutral temperature (30 °C) exceeds 140 % of normal at admission, reduces to 130 % once the wounds are fully healed, then to 120 % at 6 months after injury, and 110 % at 12–36 months post-burn [1, 25, 43, 44]. Increases in catabolism result in loss of total body protein, decreased immune defenses, and decreased wound healing [45].

2.3.3.2 Muscle Catabolism

Post-burn, muscle protein is degraded much faster than it is synthesized. Net protein loss leads to loss of lean body mass and severe muscle wasting leading to decreased strength and failure to fully rehabilitate [20, 45, 46]. Significant decreases in lean body mass related to chronic illness or hypermetabolism can have dire consequences.

10 % loss of lean body mass is associated with immune dysfunction.

20 % loss of lean body mass positively correlates with decreased wound healing.

30 % loss of lean body mass leads to increased risk for pneumonia and pressure sores.

40 % loss of lean body mass can lead to death [47].

Uncomplicated severely burned patients can lose up to 25 % of total body mass after acute burn injury [48], and protein degradation persists up to 2–3 years post severe burn injury resulting in significant negative whole-body and cross-leg nitrogen balance [20, 45, 49]. Protein catabolism has a positive correlation with increases in metabolic rates [45]. Severely burned patients have a daily nitrogen loss of 20–25 g/m^2 of burned skin [20, 45, 46]. At this rate, a lethal cachexia can be reached in less than 1 month. Burned pediatric patients' protein loss leads to significant developmental delay for up to 24–36 months post-injury [44].

Severe burn causes marked changes in body composition during acute hospitalization. Severely burned children lost about 2 % of their body weight (−5 % LBM, −3 % BMC, and −2 % BMD) from admission to discharge. Total fat and percent fat increased from admission to discharge by 3 and 7 %, respectively.

Septic patients have a particularly profound increase in metabolic rates and protein catabolism up to 40 % more compared to those with like-size burns that do not develop sepsis [45]. A vicious cycle develops, as patients that are catabolic are more susceptible to sepsis due to changes in immune function and immune response. Modulation of the hypermetabolic, hypercatabolic response thus preventing secondary injury is paramount in the restoration of structure and function of severely burned patients.

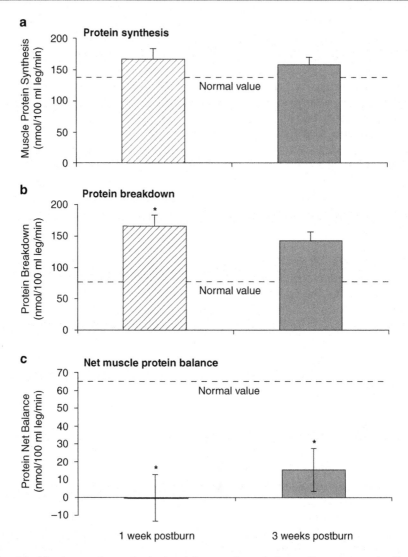

Fig. 2.3 Muscle protein synthesis, breakdown and net balance. Burn causes significant increased net protein balance was leading to catabolism. From: [1]

2.3.3.3 Glucose and Lipid Metabolism

Elevated circulating levels of catecholamines, glucagon, and cortisol after severe thermal injury stimulate free fatty acids and glycerol from fat, glucose production by the liver, and amino acids from muscle [37, 50, 51]. Specifically, glycolytic-gluconeogenic cycling is increased 250 % during the post-burn hyper-metabolic response coupled with an increase of 450 % in triglyceride-fatty acid cycling [52]. These changes lead to increased lipolysis, fatty infiltration in various organs, hyperglycemia, and impaired insulin sensitivity related to post-receptor insulin resistance and significant reductions in glucose clearance [17, 42, 53, 54].

In critical illness, metabolic alterations cause significant changes in energy substrate metabolism. In order to provide glucose, a major fuel source to vital organs, release of the above-mentioned stress mediators oppose the anabolic actions of insulin [55]. By enhancing adipose tissue lipolysis [51] and skeletal muscle proteolysis [56], they increase gluconeogenic substrates, including glycerol, alanine, and lactate, thus augmenting hepatic glucose production in burned patients [57–59]. Hyperglycemia fails to suppress hepatic glucose release during this time [60], and the suppressive effect of insulin on hepatic glucose release is attenuated, significantly contributing to post-trauma hyperglycemia [61]. Catecholamine-mediated enhancement of hepatic glycogenolysis, as well as direct sympathetic stimulation of glycogen breakdown, can further aggravate the hyperglycemia in response to stress [57]. Catecholamines have also been shown to impair glucose disposal via alterations of the insulin-signaling pathway and GLUT-4 translocation muscle and adipose tissue, resulting in peripheral insulin resistance [58, 62].

2.3.4   Renal System

Diminished blood volume and cardiac output result in decreased renal blood flow and glomerular filtration rate. Other stress-induced hormones and mediators such as angiotensin, aldosterone, and vasopressin further reduce renal blood flow immediately after the injury. These effects result in oliguria, which if left untreated will cause acute tubular necrosis and renal failure. Twenty years ago, acute renal failure in burn injuries was almost always fatal. Today newer techniques in dialysis became widely used to support the kidneys during recovery. The latest reports indicate an 88 % mortality rate for severely burned adults and a 56 % mortality rate for severely burned children in whom renal failure develops in the post-burn period [63, 64]. Early resuscitation decreases risks of renal failure and improves the associated morbidity and mortality [65].

If dialysis is needed, there are various approaches:
- Peritoneal dialysis (Tenckhoff catheter) for pediatric patients
- Hemofiltration or hemodialysis for adult patients
  We recommend using the dialysis form that is present in the individual setup.

The use of diuretics has been discussed controversially, but there seems to be strong support for the use of diuretics such as Lasix for patients being over-resuscitated, renal protection, or pulmonary edema.

2.3.5   Gastrointestinal System

The gastrointestinal response to burn is highlighted by mucosal atrophy, changes in digestive absorption, and increased intestinal permeability [66]. Atrophy of the small bowel mucosa occurs within 12 h of injury in proportion to the burn size and is related to increased epithelial cell death by apoptosis [66]. The cytoskeleton of the mucosal brush border undergoes atrophic changes associated with vesiculation of microvilli and disruption of the terminal web actin filaments. These findings were most pronounced 18 h after injury, which suggests that changes in the cytoskeleton, such as those associated with cell death by apoptosis, are processes involved in the changed gut mucosa [66]. Burn also causes reduced uptake of glucose and amino acids, decreased absorption of fatty acids, and reduction in brush border lipase activity. These changes peak in the first several hours after burn and return to normal at 48–72 h after injury, a timing that parallels mucosal atrophy.

Intestinal permeability to macromolecules, which are normally repelled by an intact mucosal barrier, increases after burn [67, 68]. Intestinal permeability to poly-ethylene glycol, lactulose, and mannitol increases after injury, correlating to the extent of the burn. Gut permeability increases even further when burn wounds become infected. A study using fluorescent dextrans showed that larger molecules appeared to cross the mucosa between the cells, whereas the smaller molecules tra-versed the mucosa through the epithelial cells, presumably by pinocytosis and vesic-ulation. Mucosal permeability also paralleled increases in gut epithelial apoptosis.

The best treatment to alleviate mucosal atrophy is early initiation of enteral nutri-tion, usually within 8–12 h post-burn. Glutamin and other antioxidants have been shown to improve enteral inflammatory-driven pathways as well as gut function.

Despite the need for liver function and integrity, the liver is profoundly affected post-burn and in our opinion a central contributor to post-burn morbidity and mortality [69–71]. The liver has several myriad functions that are each essential for survival.

All of these hepatic functions are affected by a thermal injury, and we have strong evidence that hepatic biomarkers predict and determine morbidity and mortality in severely burned patients. We, therefore, believe that the liver is central for post-burn

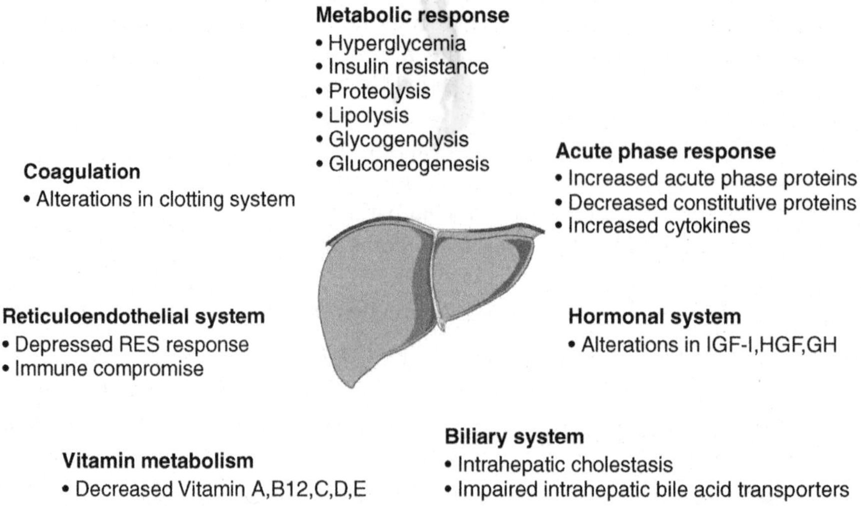

Metabolic response
- Hyperglycemia
- Insulin resistance
- Proteolysis
- Lipolysis
- Glycogenolysis
- Gluconeogenesis

Coagulation
- Alterations in clotting system

Acute phase response
- Increased acute phase proteins
- Decreased constitutive proteins
- Increased cytokines

Reticuloendothelial system
- Depressed RES response
- Immune compromise

Hormonal system
- Alterations in IGF-I,HGF,GH

Vitamin metabolism
- Decreased Vitamin A,B12,C,D,E

Biliary system
- Intrahepatic cholestasis
- Impaired intrahepatic bile acid transporters

Fig. 2.4 Multiple functions essential for out cores related to the liver from [69]

outcome, and we propose that attenuation of liver damage and restoration of liver function will improve morbidity and mortality of severely burned patients [69–71].

There is currently no treatment for hepatic dysfunction or failure post-burn. Animal and in vitro studies suggested a beneficial effect on hepatic apoptosis and function with the use of insulin and propranolol.

2.3.6 Immune System

Burns cause a global depression in immune function, which is shown by prolonged allograft skin survival on burn wounds. Burn patients are then at great risk for a number of infectious complications, including bacterial wound infection, pneumonia, and fungal and viral infections. These susceptibilities and conditions are based on depressed cellular function in all parts of the immune system, including activation and activity of neutrophils, macrophages, T lymphocytes, and B lymphocytes. With burns of more than 20 % TBSA, impairment of these immune functions is proportional to burn size.

Macrophage production after burn is diminished, which is related to the spontaneous elaboration of negative regulators of myeloid growth. This effect is enhanced by the presence of endotoxin and can be partially reversed with granulocyte colony-stimulating factor (G-CSF) treatment or inhibition of prostaglandin E_2. Investigators have shown that G-CSF levels actually increase after severe burn. However, bone marrow G-CSF receptor expression is decreased, which may in part account for the immunodeficiency seen in burns. Total neutrophil counts are initially increased after burn, a phenomenon that is related to a decrease in cell death by apoptosis. However, neutrophils that are present are dysfunctional in terms of diapedesis, chemotaxis, and phagocytosis. These effects are explained, in part, by a deficiency in CD11b/CD18 expression after inflammatory stimuli, decreased respiratory burst activity associated with a deficiency in p47-phox activity, and impaired actin mechanics related to neutrophil motile responses. After 48–72 h, neutrophil counts decrease somewhat like macrophages with similar causes.

T-helper cell function is depressed after a severe burn that is associated with polarization from the interleukin-2 and interferon-γ cytokine-based T-helper 1 (T_H1) response toward the T_H2 response. The T_H2 response is characterized by the production of interleukin-4 and interleukin-10. The T_H1 response is important in cell-mediated immune defense, whereas the T_H2 response is important in antibody responses to infection. As this polarization increases, so does the mortality rate. Burn also impairs cytotoxic T-lymphocyte activity as a function of burn size, thus increasing the risk of infection, particularly from fungi and viruses. Early burn wound excision improves cytotoxic T-cell activity.

2.4   Summary and Conclusion

Thermal injury results in massive fluid shifts from the circulating plasma into the interstitial fluid space causing hypovolemia and swelling of the burned skin. When burn injury exceeds 20–30 % TBSA, there is minimal edema generation in non-injured tissues and organs. The Starling forces change to favor fluid extravasation from blood to tissue. Rapid edema formation is predominating from the development of strongly negative interstitial fluid pressure (imbibition pressure) and to a lesser degree by an increase in microvascular pressure and permeability. Secondary to the thermal insult, there is release of inflammatory mediators and stress hormones. Circulating mediators deleteriously increase microvascular permeability and alter cellular membrane function by which water and sodium enter cells. Circulating mediators also favor renal conservation of water and salt, impair cardiac contractility, and cause vasoconstrictors, which further aggravate ischemia from combined hypovolemia and cardiac dysfunction. The end result of this complex chain of events is decreased intravascular volume, increased systemic vascular resistance, decreased cardiac output, end-organ ischemia, and metabolic acidosis. Early excision of the devitalized tissue appears to reduce the local and systemic effects of mediators released from burned tissue, thus reducing the progressive pathophysiologic derangements. Without early and full resuscitation therapy, these derangements can result in acute renal failure, vascular ischemia, cardiovascular collapse, and death. Edema in both the burn wound and particularly in the non-injured soft tissue is increased by resuscitation. Edema is a serious complication, which likely contributes to decreased tissue oxygen diffusion and further ischemic insult to already damaged cells with compromised blood flow increasing the risk of infection. Research should continue to focus on methods to ameliorate the severe edema and vasoconstriction that exacerbate tissue ischemia. The success of this research will require identification of key circulatory factors that alter capillary permeability, cause vasoconstriction, depolarize cellular membranes, and depress myocardial function. Hopefully, methods to prevent the release and to block the activity of specific mediators can be further developed in order to reduce the morbidity and mortality rates of burn shock. The profound and overall metabolic alterations post-burn associated with persistent changes in glucose metabolism and impaired insulin sensitivity also significantly contribute to adverse outcome of this patient population and constitute another challenge for future therapeutic approaches of this unique patient population.

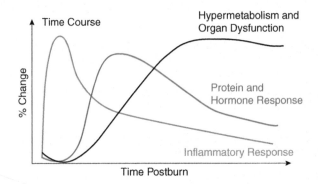

of various responses contributing to post-burn morbidity and mortality

References

1. Jeschke MG, Chinkes DL, Finnerty CC et al (2008) Pathophysiologic response to severe burn injury. Ann Surg 248(3):387–401
2. Herndon DN (2007) Total burn care, 3rd edn. Saunders Elsevier, Philadelphia
3. Jeschke MG, Kamolz L, Sjoeberg F, Wolf SE (2012) Handbook of burns, vol 1. Springer, Wien/New York
4. Berger MM (2005) Can oxidative damage be treated nutritionally? Clin Nutr (Edinburgh, Scotland) 24:172–183
5. Berger MM (2006) Antioxidant micronutrients in major trauma and burns: evidence and practice. Nutr Clin Pract 21:438–449
6. Jeschke MG, Rose C, Angele P, Fuchtmeier B, Nerlich MN, Bolder U (2004) Development of new reconstructive techniques: use of Integra in combination with fibrin glue and negative-pressure therapy for reconstruction of acute and chronic wounds. Plast Reconstr Surg 113:525–530
7. Demling RH, DeSanti L (2001) The rate of restoration of body weight after burn injury, using the anabolic agent oxandrolone, is not age dependent. Burns 27:46–51
8. Demling RH, Seigne P (2000) Metabolic management of patients with severe burns. World J Surg 24:673–680
9. Branski LK, Herndon DN, Byrd JF et al (2011) Transpulmonary thermodilution for hemodynamic measurements in severely burned children. Crit Care 15:R118
10. Kraft R, Herndon DN, Branski LK, Finnerty CC, Leonard KR, Jeschke MG (2012) Optimized fluid management improves outcomes of pediatric burn patients. J Surg Res 2012 June 6 Epub first
11. Williams FN, Herndon DN, Suman OE et al (2011) Changes in cardiac physiology after severe burn injury. J Burn Care Res 32:269–274
12. Wilmore DW, Long JM, Mason AD Jr, Skreen RW, Pruitt BA Jr (1974) Catecholamines: mediator of the hypermetabolic response to thermal injury. Ann Surg 180:653–669
13. Arturson G (1961) Pathophysiological aspects of the burn syndrome with special reference to liver injury and alterations of capillary permeability. Acta Chir Scand Suppl 274(Suppl):1–135
14. Demling RH, Mazess RB, Witt RM, Wolberg WH (1978) The study of burn wound edema using dichromatic absorptiometry. J Trauma 18:124–128
15. Demling RH, Will JA, Belzer FO (1978) Effect of major thermal injury on the pulmonary microcirculation. Surgery 83:746–751
16. Leape LL (1970) Initial changes in burns: tissue changes in burned and unburned skin of rhesus monkeys. J Trauma 10:488–492
17. Wilmore DW (1976) Hormonal responses and their effect on metabolism. Surg Clin North Am 56:999–1018
18. Cuthbertson DP, Angeles Valero Zanuy MA, Leon Sanz ML (2001) Post-shock metabolic response 1942. Nutr Hosp 16:176–182; discussion 5–6
19. Baron PW, Barrow RE, Pierre EJ, Herndon DN (1997) Prolonged use of propranolol safely decreases cardiac work in burned children. J Burn Care Rehabil 18:223–227
20. Herndon DN, Tompkins RG (2004) Support of the metabolic response to burn injury. Lancet 363:1895–1902
21. Minifee PK, Barrow RE, Abston S, Desai M, Herndon DN (1989) Improved myocardial oxygen utilization following propranolol infusion in adolescents with postburn hypermetabolism. J Pediatr Surg 24:806–810; discussion 10–11
22. Horton JW (2004) Left ventricular contractile dysfunction as a complication of thermal injury. Shock 22:495–507
23. Horton JW, White DJ, Maass D, Sanders B, Thompson M, Giroir B (1999) Calcium antagonists improve cardiac mechanical performance after thermal trauma. J Surg Res 87:39–50

24. Jeschke MG, Mlcak RP, Finnerty CC et al (2007) Burn size determines the inflammatory and hypermetabolic response. Crit Care 11:R90

25. Hart DW, Wolf SE, Mlcak R et al (2000) Persistence of muscle catabolism after severe burn. Surgery 128:312–319

26. Mlcak RP, Jeschke MG, Barrow RE, Herndon DN (2006) The influence of age and gender on resting energy expenditure in severely burned children. Ann Surg 244:121–130

27. Przkora R, Barrow RE, Jeschke MG et al (2006) Body composition changes with time in pediatric burn patients. J Trauma 60:968–971; discussion 71

28. Przkora R, Herndon DN, Suman OE (2007) The effects of oxandrolone and exercise on muscle mass and function in children with severe burns. Pediatrics 119:e109–e116

29. Dolecek R (1989) Endocrine changes after burn trauma – a review. Keio J Med 38:262–276

30. Jeffries MK, Vance ML (1992) Growth hormone and cortisol secretion in patients with burn injury. J Burn Care Rehabil 13:391–395

31. Klein GL, Bi LX, Sherrard DJ et al (2004) Evidence supporting a role of glucocorticoids in short-term bone loss in burned children. Osteoporos Int 15:468–474

32. Goodall M, Stone C, Haynes BW Jr (1957) Urinary output of adrenaline and noradrenaline in severe thermal burns. Ann Surg 145:479–487

33. Coombes EJ, Batstone GF (1982) Urine cortisol levels after burn injury. Burns Incl Therm Inj 8:333–337

34. Norbury WB, Herndon DN (2007) Modulation of the hypermetabolic response after burn injury. In: Herndon DN (ed) Total burn care, 3rd edn. Saunders Elsevier, New York, pp 420–433

35. Sheridan RL (2001) A great constitutional disturbance. N Engl J Med 345:1271–1272

36. Pereira C, Murphy K, Jeschke M, Herndon DN (2005) Post burn muscle wasting and the effects of treatments. Int J Biochem Cell Biol 37:1948–1961

37. Wolfe RR (1981) Review: acute versus chronic response to burn injury. Circ Shock 8:105–115

38. Galster AD, Bier DM, Cryer PE, Monafo WW (1984) Plasma palmitate turnover in subjects with thermal injury. J Trauma 24:938–945

39. Cree MG, Zwetsloot JJ, Herndon DN et al (2007) Insulin sensitivity and mitochondrial function are improved in children with burn injury during a randomized controlled trial of fenofibrate. Ann Surg 245:214–221

40. Childs C, Heath DF, Little RA, Brotherston M (1990) Glucose metabolism in children during the first day after burn injury. Arch Emerg Med 7:135–147

41. Cree MG, Aarsland A, Herndon DN, Wolfe RR (2007) Role of fat metabolism in burn trauma-induced skeletal muscle insulin resistance. Crit Care Med 35:S476–S483

42. Gauglitz GG, Herndon DN, Kulp GA, Meyer WJ 3rd, Jeschke MG (2009) Abnormal insulin sensitivity persists up to three years in pediatric patients post-burn. J Clin Endocrinol Metabol 94:1656–1664

43. Hart DW, Wolf SE, Herndon DN et al (2002) Energy expenditure and caloric balance after burn: increased feeding leads to fat rather than lean mass accretion. Ann Surg 235:152–161

44. Jeschke MG, Gauglitz GG, Kulp GA et al (2011) Long-term persistence of the pathophysiologic response to severe burn injury. PLoS One 6:e21245

45. Hart DW, Wolf SE, Chinkes DL et al (2000) Determinants of skeletal muscle catabolism after severe burn. Ann Surg 232:455–465

46. Herndon DN, Hart DW, Wolf SE, Chinkes DL, Wolfe RR (2001) Reversal of catabolism by beta-blockade after severe burns. N Engl J Med 345:1223–1229

47. Chang DW, DeSanti L, Demling RH (1998) Anticatabolic and anabolic strategies in critical illness: a review of current treatment modalities. Shock 10:155–160

48. Newsome TW, Mason ADJ, Pruitt BAJ (1973) Weight loss following thermal injury. Ann Surg 178:215–217

49. Jahoor F, Desai M, Herndon DN, Wolfe RR (1988) Dynamics of the protein metabolic response to burn injury. Metabolism 37:330–337
50. Wolfe RR, Shaw JH, Durkot MJ (1983) Energy metabolism in trauma and sepsis: the role of fat. Prog Clin Biol Res 111:89–109
51. Wolfe RR, Herndon DN, Jahoor F, Miyoshi H, Wolfe M (1987) Effect of severe burn injury on substrate cycling by glucose and fatty acids. N Engl J Med 317:403–408
52. Yu YM, Tompkins RG, Ryan CM, Young VR (1999) The metabolic basis of the increase of the increase in energy expenditure in severely burned patients. JPEN J Parenter Enteral Nutr 23:160–168
53. Gauglitz GG, Herndon DN, Jeschke MG (2008) Insulin resistance postburn: underlying mechanisms and current therapeutic strategies. J Burn Care Res 29:683–694
54. Gauglitz GG, Halder S, Boehning DF et al (2010) Post-burn hepatic insulin resistance is associated with Er stress. Shock 33(3):299–305
55. Khani S, Tayek JA (2001) Cortisol increases gluconeogenesis in humans: its role in the metabolic syndrome. Clin Sci (Lond) 101:739–747
56. Gore DC, Jahoor F, Wolfe RR, Herndon DN (1993) Acute response of human muscle protein to catabolic hormones. Ann Surg 218:679–684
57. Robinson LE, van Soeren MH (2004) Insulin resistance and hyperglycemia in critical illness: role of insulin in glycemic control. AACN Clin Issues 15:45–62
58. Gearhart MM, Parbhoo SK (2006) Hyperglycemia in the critically ill patient. AACN Clin Issues 17:50–55
59. Carlson GL (2001) Insulin resistance and glucose-induced thermogenesis in critical illness. Proc Nutr Soc 60:381–388
60. Wolfe RR, Durkot MJ, Allsop JR, Burke JF (1979) Glucose metabolism in severely burned patients. Metabolism 28:1031–1039
61. Cree MG, Wolfe RR (2008) Postburn trauma insulin resistance and fat metabolism. Am J Physiol Endocrinol Metab 294:E1–E9
62. Hunt DG, Ivy JL (2002) Epinephrine inhibits insulin-stimulated muscle glucose transport. J Appl Physiol 93:1638–1643
63. Chrysopoulo MT, Jeschke MG, Dziewulski P, Barrow RE, Herndon DN (1999) Acute renal dysfunction in severely burned adults. J Trauma 46:141–144
64. Jeschke MG, Barrow RE, Wolf SE, Herndon DN (1998) Mortality in burned children with acute renal failure. Arch Surg 133:752–756
65. Wolf SE, Rose JK, Desai MH, Mileski JP, Barrow RE, Herndon DN (1997) Mortality determinants in massive pediatric burns. An analysis of 103 children with > or=80 % TBSA burns (> or=70 % full-thickness). Ann Surg 225:554–565; discussion 65–69
66. Wolf SE, Ikeda H, Matin S et al (1999) Cutaneous burn increases apoptosis in the gut epithelium of mice. J Am Coll Surg 188:10–16
67. Deitch EA, Rutan R, Waymack JP (1996) Trauma, shock, and gut translocation. New Horiz 4:289–299
68. Swank GM, Deitch EA (1996) Role of the gut in multiple organ failure: bacterial translocation and permeability changes. World J Surg 20:411–417
69. Jeschke MG (2009) The hepatic response to thermal injury: is the liver important for postburn outcomes? Mol Med 15(9-10):337–351
70. Jeschke MG, Barrow RE, Herndon DN (2004) Extended hypermetabolic response of the liver in severely burned pediatric patients. Arch Surg 139:641–647
71. Jeschke MG, Mlcak RP, Herndon DN (2007) Morphologic changes of the liver after a severe thermal injury. Shock Aug 28(2):172–177

Wound Healing and Wound Care

Gerd G. Gauglitz

3.1 Introduction

Understanding a burn injury and its associated complex wound-healing cascade requires recognition of the anatomy and physiology of the skin. The skin is a bilayer organ with many protective functions essential for survival.

- The outer epidermal layer provides critical barrier functions and is composed of an outer layer of dead cells and keratin, which present a barrier to bacterial and environmental toxins.
- The basal epidermal cells supply the source of new epidermal cells. The undulating surface of the epidermis, called rete pegs, increases adherence of the epidermis to the dermis via the basement membrane.
- The inner dermal layer has a number of essential functions, including continued restoration of the epidermis.
- The dermis is divided into the papillary dermis and the reticular dermis. The former is extremely bioactive; the latter, less bioactive. This difference in bioactivity within the dermis is the reason that superficial partial-thickness burns generally heal faster than deeper partial-thickness burns; the papillary component is lost in the deeper burns.
- Loss of and damage to the normal skin barrier function causes the common complications of burn injury. These include:
  - Infection
  - Loss of body heat
  - Increased evaporative water loss
  - Change in key interactive functions such as touch and appearance
  - Excessive scarring leading to contractures

G.G. Gauglitz, MMS, MD
Department of Dermatology and Allergology,
Ludwig Maximilians University,
Frauenlobstr. 9-11, 80337 Munich, Germany
e-mail: gerd.gauglitz@med.uni-muenchen.de

M.G. Jeschke et al. (eds.), *Burn Care and Treatment*,
DOI 10.1007/978-3-7091-1133-8_3, © Springer-Verlag Wien 2013

- Scars form as a result of the physiologic wound-healing process and may arise following any insult to the deep dermis.
- Genetic susceptibility, specific anatomic locations, prolonged inflammation, and delayed epithelialization significantly increase the risk of developing excessive scarring.
- Hypertrophic scarring forms frequently after burn injury with incidence rates varying from 40 to up to 91 %, depending on the depth of the wound [1, 2].

3.2 Physiological Versus Pathophysiologic Wound Healing

The physiologic response to wounding in adult tissue is the formation of a scar and can be temporally grouped into three distinct phases:
- Inflammation
- Proliferation
- Remodeling [3–5]
- Immediately following wounding, platelet degranulation and activation of the complement and clotting cascades form a fibrin clot for hemostasis, which acts as a scaffold for wound repair [3].
- Platelet degranulation is responsible for the release and activation of an array of potent cytokines, such as epidermal growth factor (EGF), insulin-like growth factor (IGF-I), platelet-derived growth factor (PDGF), and transforming growth factor beta (TGF-β), which serve as chemotactic agents for the recruitment of neutrophils, macrophages, epithelial cells, mast cells, endothelial cells, and fibroblasts [3, 6].
- Forty-eight to 72 h after the initial event, the healing process transitions into the *proliferation phase* which may last for up to 3–6 weeks [7]. Recruited fibroblasts synthesize a scaffold of reparative tissue, the so-called extracellular matrix (ECM). This granulation tissue is made of procollagen, elastin, proteoglycans, and hyaluronic acid and forms a structural repair framework to bridge the wound and allow vascular ingrowth [7]. Modified fibroblasts, so-called myofibroblasts, containing actin filaments help in initiating wound contraction.
- Once the wound is closed, the immature scar can transition into the *final maturation phase*, which may last several months. The abundant ECM is then degraded, and the immature type III collagen of the early wound can be modified into mature type I collagen [7].
- *The transformation of a wound clot into granulation tissue thus requires a delicate balance between ECM protein deposition and degradation, and when disrupted, abnormalities in scarring appear, resulting in excessive scar formation [5].*
- Recent evidence suggests that it is not simply the severity of inflammation that predisposes to excessive scarring but also the type of the immune response [8]. T-helper cells (CD41) cells have been implicated as major immunoregulators in wound healing.
- The characteristic cytokine expression profile of the CD41 T cells represents the basis for describing either a predominantly Th1 or Th2 response to a specific or unspecific stimulus [5, 9].

- While the development of a Th2 response (with production of interleukin (IL)-4, IL-5, IL-10, and IL-13) has been strongly linked to fibrogenesis, a predominance of Th1 CD41 cells has been shown to almost completely attenuate the formation of tissue fibrosis via production of interferon gamma (IFN-γ) and IL-12 [10, 11].

3.2.1 Transforming Growth Factor Beta

Many of the biologic actions of TGF-β contribute to the normal wound-healing process and have been implicated in a wide variety of fibrotic disorders [5]. Early after injury, high levels of TGF-β are being released from degranulating platelets at the site of injury, where they act as chemoattractants for lymphocytes, fibroblasts, monocytes, and neutrophils [12].

- The TGF-β family consists of at least five highly conserved polypeptides, with TGF-β1, TGF-β2, and TGF-β3 being the principal mammalian forms.
- *TGF-β1 and TGF-β2 are one of the most important stimulators of collagen and proteoglycan synthesis, and affects the ECM not only by stimulating collagen synthesis but also by preventing its breakdown* [13, 14].
- *TGF-β3, which is predominantly induced in the later stages of wound healing, has been found to reduce connective tissue deposition* [15].
- *Specifically, beyond 1 week, differential expression of TGF-β isoforms, receptors, and activity modulators, rather than the mere presence or absence of TGF-β, may have a major role in the development of both, keloids and hypertrophic scarring* [16].

3.2.2 Interactions Between Keratinocytes and Fibroblasts

Keratinocytes have been shown to mediate the behavior of fibroblasts during wound healing through their secretion, activation, or inhibition of growth factors such as TGF-β [9]. Particularly, release of IL-1 from keratinocytes at the wound site seems to represent the initial trigger for the inflammatory reaction and serves as an autocrine signal to fibroblasts and endothelial cells, resulting in a pleiotropic effect on them [17, 18].

3.2.3 Matrix Metalloproteinases (MMP)

The major effectors of ECM degradation and remodeling belong to a family of structurally related enzymes called MMP [5]. The MMP family consists of about 25 zinc-dependent and calcium-dependent proteinases in the mammalian system [19].

- An imbalance in expression of MMPs has been implicated in a number of pathological conditions such as dermal fibrosis [20], tumor invasion, and metastasis [21].
- Several MMPs have been shown to mediate the breakdown of types I and III collagen, the most abundant types of collagen in the skin ECM [19]. Specifically,

MMP-2 and MMP-9 activity persists after wound closure and seems to play a potent role in the remodeling process [22].

3.3   Wound Care Post-Burn

Treatment of burn wounds depends on the characteristics and size of the wound. All treatments are aimed at rapid and painless healing. Current therapy directed specifically toward burn wounds can be divided into three stages: assessment, management, and rehabilitation.
- Once the extent and depth of the wounds have been assessed and the wounds have been thoroughly cleaned and débrided, the management phase begins.
- Each wound should be dressed with an appropriate covering that serves several functions. First, it should protect the damaged epithelium, minimize bacterial and fungal colonization, and provide splinting action to maintain the desired position of function.
- Second, the dressing should be occlusive to reduce evaporative heat loss and minimize cold stress.
- Third, the dressing should provide comfort over the painful wound.
  The choice of dressing is based on the characteristics of the treated wound:
- First-degree wounds are minor with minimal loss of barrier function. These wounds require no dressing and are treated with topical salves to decrease pain and keep the skin moist.
- Second-degree wounds can be treated with daily dressing changes with topical antibiotics, cotton gauze, and elastic wraps. Alternatively, the wounds can be treated with a temporary biological or synthetic covering to close the wound.
- Deep second-degree and third-degree wounds require excision and grafting for sizable burns, and the choice of initial dressing should be aimed at holding bacterial proliferation in check and providing occlusion until the operation is performed.

3.3.1   Burn Wound Excision

Methods for handling burn wounds have changed in recent decades and are similar in adults and children.
- Increasingly aggressive early tangential excision of the burn tissue and early wound closure primarily by skin grafts have led to significant improvement of mortality rates and substantially lower costs in this particular patient population [23–27].
- Early wound closure has been furthermore found to be associated with decreased severity of hypertrophic scarring, joint contractures, and stiffness and promotes quicker rehabilitation [23, 26].
- In general most areas are excised with a hand skin graft knife or powered dermatome.

- Sharp excision with a knife or electrocautery is reserved for areas of functional cosmetic importance such as hand and face.
- In partial-thickness wounds, an attempt is being made to preserve viable dermis, whereas in full-thickness injury, all necrotic and infected tissue must be removed leaving a viable wound bed of either fascia, fat, or muscle [28].

3.3.2 Burn Wound Coverage

Following burn wound excision, it is vital to obtain wound closure. Various biological and synthetic substrates have been employed to replace the injured skin post-burn.

3.3.3 Autografts

Autografts from uninjured skin remain the mainstay of treatment for many patients. Since early wound closure using autograft may be difficult when full-thickness burns exceed 40 % total body surface area (TBSA), *allografts* (cadaver skin) frequently serve as skin substitute in severely burned patients. While this approach is still commonly used in burn centers throughout the world, it bears considerable risks, including antigenicity, cross-infection, as well as limited availability [29]. *Xenografts* have been used for hundreds of years as temporary replacement for skin loss. Even though these grafts provide a biologically active dermal matrix, the immunologic disparities prevent engraftment and predetermine rejection over time [30]. However, both xenografts and allografts are only a mean of temporary burn wound cover. True closure can only be achieved with living autografts or isografts.

3.3.4 Epidermal Substitutes

Autologous epithelial cells grown from a single full-thickness skin biopsy have been available for nearly two decades. These cultured epithelial autografts (CEA) have shown to decrease mortality in massively burned patients in a prospective, controlled trial [31]. However, widespread use of cultured epithelial autografts has been primarily hampered by poor long-term clinical results, exorbitant costs, and fragility and difficult handling of these grafts, which have been consistently reported by different burn units treating deep burns, even when cells were applied on properly prepared wound beds [30, 32, 33].

- Currently commercially available autologous epidermal substitutes for clinical use include CellSpray (Clinical Cell Culture (C3), Perth, Australia), Epicel (Genzyme Biosurgery, Cambridge, MA, USA), EpiDex (Modex Therapeutiques, Lausanne, Switzerland), and Bioseed-S (BioTissue Technologies GmbH, Freiburg, Germany).

- There have been several studies testing epithelial allografts [34–36]; however, controlled clinical studies confirming the effectiveness and safety of these products are needed. Alternatively, dermal analogs have been made available for clinical use in recent years.

3.3.5   Dermal Substitutes

In contrast to cultured epidermal sheets, engineered dermal constructs can prevent wound contraction, and they provide a greater mechanical stability. To date, a wide variety of marketed dermal constructs is available. These skin substitutes can promote the healing of acute and chronic wounds [37] by secreting extracellular matrix (ECM) proteins, a variety of growth factors, and cytokines into the wound until they undergo normal apoptosis a few weeks postimplantation [38]. An overview summarizing commercially available dermal constructs for clinical use is given in Table 3.1.

- Some of these substitutes are chemically treated allografts (e.g., Alloderm®), lacking the cellular elements that are responsible for the immunogenic rejection [39].
- Dermagraft® (Advanced Biohealing; La Jolla, CA) consists of human foreskin fibroblasts, cultured in a biodegradable polyglactin mesh [40, 41]. It stimulates ingrowth of fibrovascular tissue and epithelialization. The frozen product offers an advantage but unfortunately requires storage at −75 °C. It is thawed in sterile saline and then applied to a clean, well-debrided wound. It has a 6-month shelf life and was approved by the FDA in 2001 for full-thickness diabetic foot ulcers of more than 6 weeks' duration, extending through the dermis, but without exposed underlying structures. It has found value in healing complex surgical wounds with secondary closure.
- Integra® was developed in 1981 and approved by the FDA in 2002. It is a bilaminar skin equivalent composed of porous matrix of cross-linked bovine collagen and shark-derived glycosaminoglycan, attached to a semipermeable silicone layer that serves as an epidermis. The membrane helps prevent water loss and provides a flexible wound covering, while the scaffolding promotes neovascularization and new dermal growth. Cells migrate into the matrix, while the bovine collagen is absorbed and replaced by the patient's dermal elements. Rebuilding of the scaffolding occurs within 2–3 weeks, at which time the silicone layer is removed, allowing reepithelialization from the wound edge. Complete wound closure takes approximately 30 days. Indications for Integra include pressure, diabetic, chronic vascular, and venous ulcers, as well as surgical wounds and has been successfully utilized in immediate and delayed closure of full-thickness burns, leading to reduction in length of hospital stay, favorable cosmetics, and improved functional outcome in a prospective and controlled clinical study [42–45]. Our group recently conducted a randomized clinical trial utilizing Integra® in the management of severe full-thickness burns of ≥50 % TBSA in a pediatric patient population

Table 3.1 Commercially available dermal constructs for clinical use

Brand name	Manufacturer	Cell-free	Cell-based	Cell-seeded scaffold (TE)
AlloDerm	LifeCell Corporation, Branchburg, NJ, USA	x		–
Karoderm	Karocell Tissue Engineering AB, Karolinska University Hospital, Stockholm, Sweden	x		–
SureDerm	HANS BIOMED Corporation, Seoul, Korea	x		–
GraftJacket	Wright Medical Technology, Inc., Arlington, TN, USA	x		–
Matriderm	Dr Suwelack Skin and HealthCare AG, Billerbeck, Germany	x		–
Permacol surgical implant	Tissue Science Laboratories plc, Aldershot, UK	x		–
OASIS Wound Matrix	Cook Biotech Inc., West Lafayette, IN, USA	x		–
EZ Derm	Brennen Medical, Inc., MN, USA	x		–
Integra Dermal Regeneration Template	Integra NeuroSciences, Plainsboro, NJ, USA	x		–
Terudermis	Olympus Terumo Biomaterial Corp., Tokyo, Japan	x		–
Pelnac Standard/ Pelnac Fortified	Gunze Ltd, Medical Materials Center, Kyoto, Japan	x		–
Biobrane/ Biobrane-L	UDL Laboratories, Inc., Rockford, IL, USA	x		–
Hyalomatrix PA	Fidia Advanced Biopolymers, Abano Terme, Italy	x		–
TransCyte (DermagraftTC)	Advanced BioHealing, Inc., New York, NY and La Jolla, CA, USA			Neonatal allogeneic fibroblasts
Dermagraft	Advanced BioHealing, Inc., New York, NY and La Jolla, CA, USA			Neonatal allogeneic fibroblasts
Hyalograft 3D	Fidia Advanced Biopolymers, Abano Terme, Italy			Autologous fibroblasts

x = applicable meaning cell-free wound coverage
Modified from Ref. [38]

comparing it to standard autograft-allograft technique and found Integra to be associated with improved resting energy expenditure and improved aesthetic outcome post-burn [46]. It has been also found to inhibit scar formation and wound contraction [47].

- Biobrane®, a temporary synthetic dressing composed of nylon mesh bonded to a silicone membrane, helps control water loss and reepithelialization [48].

3.3.6   Epidermal/Dermal Substitutes

To date, the most advanced and sophisticated constructs that are available for clinical use represent substitutes that mimic both epidermal as well as dermal layers of the skin.

- Currently available epidermal/dermal substitutes that are in clinical use include Apligraf (Organogenesis Inc., Canton, Massachusetts, CA, USA), OrCel® (Ortec International, Inc., New York, NY, USA), PolyActive® (HC Implants BV, Leiden, The Netherlands), and TissueTech® Autograft System (Laserskin and Hyalograft 3D; Fidia Advanced Biopolymers, Abano Terme, Italy). These constructs are composed of autologous and allogeneic skin cells (keratinocytes and fibroblasts), which are incorporated into scaffolds.
- Apligraf® was the first commercially available composite tissue analog on the market. This medical device containing living allogeneic cells was approved by the US Food and Drug Administration (FDA) in 1998 for the treatment of venous ulcers of 1 month's duration that have not responded to conventional therapy. It was approved in 2000 for neuropathic diabetic ulcers of more than 3 weeks' duration [49]. The epidermal component of this bilayer skin construct consists of neonatal foreskin keratinocytes seeded on a dermal component comprised of neonatal foreskin fibroblasts within a matrix of bovine type I collagen. This 0.75-cm disc has a 10-day shelf life and requires storage at 68 to 73 °F. It is secured to the prepared wound bed with sutures or a dressing and is changed weekly. Apligraf® was shown to achieve significantly better results in healing large, deep venous ulcers of more than 1 year's duration when compared to compression [50]. Apligraf® has been also successfully used in acute surgical wounds [49] and may result in a more pliable and less vascular scar when used in wounds that would otherwise be allowed to heal with secondary intention [51].
- Orocel®, the first biologic cellular matrix, was initially developed in 1971 as a treatment for dystrophic epidermolysis bullosa [52]. Similar to Apligraf®, neonatal foreskin epidermal keratinocytes and dermal fibroblasts are cultured onto a preformed porous sponge. However, it is produced in a cryopreserved format, in contrast to the fresh product of Apligraf®.

Importantly, although mimicking the histoarchitecture of normal skin, epidermal/dermal skin substitutes should be considered as temporary biologically active wound dressings [40]. Composite skin substitutes have been shown to provide growth factors, cytokines, and ECM for host cells, and by that, initiating and regulating wound healing. Nevertheless, these skin substitutes are accompanied by high manufacturing costs and repeatedly fail to close the wound permanently due to tissue rejection [38].

Advances in stem cell culture technology may represent another promising therapeutic approach to deliver cosmetic restoration for burn patients.

3.3.7 Stem Cell-Based Therapies

Encouraging results from stem cell-based treatment strategies in post-infarction myocardial repair [53] have led to application of similar strategies in order to treat skin wounds, where positive effects on all phases of wound healing have been reported with various types of mesenchymal stem cells (MSC) [54–60]. In addition, the implantation of hair follicles (HFs) in Integra® skin equivalent templates for transplantation onto a human patient's burn wound accelerated reepithelialization, minimized skin graft failure by reconstituting the epithelial stem cell pool, and was felt to produce cosmetically satisfactory results [60]. Other than transplantation, recruiting endogenous stem cells to the site of injury presents an alternative for the treatment of cutaneous wounds [61, 62].

However, several issues need to be considered before administering stem cells to wound patients:

- Functionality of stem cells decreases with age, thus older patients may not present the perfect population as donors [63–65].
- The risk of immunological rejection upon transplant or transfusion must be considered if using stem cells from allogeneic sources.

3.4 Summary

Loss of the normal skin barrier function causes the common complications of burn injury. These include infection, loss of body heat, increased evaporative water loss, and change in key interactive functions such as touch and appearance. Excessive scar formation in the areas of a deep dermal burn represents an additional well-known side effect that significantly affects the patient's quality of life, both physically and psychologically.

Early excision and early closure of the burn wound has been probably the single greatest advancement in the treating patients with severe thermal injuries during the last 20 years. Despite all efforts, an off-the-shelf, full-thickness skin replacement is not yet available. A future prospective is to incorporate cellular growth-enhancing substances or additional cell types, besides keratinocytes and fibroblasts, in the bioengineered skin substitutes to obtain constructs with improved function and higher resemblance to native skin. The development of gene transfer technology and the use of stem cells appear to be a promising means in this context.

References

1. Deitch EA, Wheelahan TM, Rose MP, Clothier J, Cotter J (1983) Hypertrophic burn scars: analysis of variables. J Trauma 23(10):895–898

2. Lewis WH, Sun KK (1990) Hypertrophic scar: a genetic hypothesis. Burns 16(3):176–178
3. Tredget EE, Nedelec B, Scott PG, Ghahary A (1997) Hypertrophic scars, keloids, and contractures. The cellular and molecular basis for therapy. Surg Clin North Am 77(3):701–730
4. Gauglitz GG, Pavicic T (2012) Emerging strategies for the prevention and therapy of excessive scars. MMW Fortschr Med 154(15):55–58
5. Gauglitz GG, Korting HC, Pavicic T, Ruzicka T, Jeschke MG (2011) Hypertrophic scarring and keloids: pathomechanisms and current and emerging treatment strategies. Mol Med 17(1–2):113–125
6. Niessen FB, Spauwen PH, Schalkwijk J, Kon M (1999) On the nature of hypertrophic scars and keloids: a review. Plast Reconstr Surg 104(5):1435–1458
7. Slemp AE, Kirschner RE (2006) Keloids and scars: a review of keloids and scars, their pathogenesis, risk factors, and management. Curr Opin Pediatr 18(4):396–402
8. Brown JJ, Bayat A (2009) Genetic susceptibility to raised dermal scarring. Br J Dermatol 161(1):8–18
9. Armour A, Scott PG, Tredget EE (2007) Cellular and molecular pathology of HTS: basis for treatment. Wound Repair Regen 15(Suppl 1):S6–S17
10. Wynn TA (2004) Fibrotic disease and the T(H)1/T(H)2 paradigm. Nat Rev Immunol 4(8):583–594
11. Doucet C, Brouty-Boye D, Pottin-Clemenceau C, Canonica GW, Jasmin C, Azzarone B (1998) Interleukin (IL) 4 and IL-13 act on human lung fibroblasts. Implication in asthma. J Clin Invest 101(10):2129–2139
12. Bullard KM, Longaker MT, Lorenz HP (2003) Fetal wound healing: current biology. World J Surg 27(1):54–61
13. Szulgit G, Rudolph R, Wandel A, Tenenhaus M, Panos R, Gardner H (2002) Alterations in fibroblast alpha1beta1 integrin collagen receptor expression in keloids and hypertrophic scars. J Invest Dermatol 118(3):409–415
14. Kose O, Waseem A (2008) Keloids and hypertrophic scars: are they two different sides of the same coin? Dermatol Surg 34(3):336–346
15. Bock O, Yu H, Zitron S, Bayat A, Ferguson MW, Mrowietz U (2005) Studies of transforming growth factors beta 1–3 and their receptors I and II in fibroblast of keloids and hypertrophic scars. Acta Derm Venereol 85(3):216–220
16. Lu L, Saulis AS, Liu WR, Roy NK, Chao JD, Ledbetter S, Mustoe TA (2005) The temporal effects of anti-TGF-beta1, 2, and 3 monoclonal antibody on wound healing and hypertrophic scar formation. J Am Coll Surg 201(3):391–397
17. Niessen FB, Schalkwijk J, Vos H, Timens W (2004) Hypertrophic scar formation is associated with an increased number of epidermal Langerhans cells. J Pathol 202(1):121–129
18. Andriessen MP, Niessen FB, Van de Kerkhof PC, Schalkwijk J (1998) Hypertrophic scarring is associated with epidermal abnormalities: an immunohistochemical study. J Pathol 186(2):192–200
19. Ghahary A, Ghaffari A (2007) Role of keratinocyte-fibroblast cross-talk in development of hypertrophic scar. Wound Repair Regen 15(Suppl 1):S46–S53
20. Ghahary A, Shen YJ, Nedelec B, Wang R, Scott PG, Tredget EE (1996) Collagenase production is lower in post-burn hypertrophic scar fibroblasts than in normal fibroblasts and is reduced by insulin-like growth factor-1. J Invest Dermatol 106(3):476–481
21. Birkedal-Hansen H, Moore WG, Bodden MK, Windsor LJ, Birkedal-Hansen B, DeCarlo A, Engler JA (1993) Matrix metalloproteinases: a review. Crit Rev Oral Biol Med 4(2):197–250
22. Fujiwara M, Muragaki Y, Ooshima A (2005) Keloid-derived fibroblasts show increased secretion of factors involved in collagen turnover and depend on matrix metalloproteinase for migration. Br J Dermatol 153(2):295–300
23. Atiyeh BS, Dham R, Kadry M, Abdallah AF, Al-Oteify M, Fathi O, Samir A (2002) Benefit-cost analysis of moist exposed burn ointment. Burns 28(7):659–663
24. Lofts JA (1991) Cost analysis of a major burn. N Z Med J 104(924):488–490
25. Munster AM, Smith-Meek M, Sharkey P (1994) The effect of early surgical intervention on mortality and cost-effectiveness in burn care, 1978–91. Burns 20(1):61–64

26. Ramzy PI, Barret JP, Herndon DN (1999) Thermal injury. Crit Care Clin 15(2):333–352, ix
27. Chan BP, Kochevar IE, Redmond RW (2002) Enhancement of porcine skin graft adherence using a light-activated process. J Surg Res 108(1):77–84
28. Dziewulski P, Barret JP (1999) Assesment, operative planning and surgery for burn wound closure. In: Wolf SE, Herndon DN (eds) Burn care. Landes Bioscience, Austin, pp 19–52
29. Blome-Eberwein S, Jester A, Kuentscher M, Raff T, Germann G, Pelzer M (2002) Clinical practice of glycerol preserved allograft skin coverage. Burns 28(Suppl 1):S10–S12
30. Garfein ES, Orgill DP, Pribaz JJ (2003) Clinical applications of tissue engineered constructs. Clin Plast Surg 30(4):485–498
31. Munster AM (1996) Cultured skin for massive burns. A prospective, controlled trial. Ann Surg 224(3):372–375; discussion 375–377
32. Bannasch H, Fohn M, Unterberg T, Bach AD, Weyand B, Stark GB (2003) Skin tissue engineering. Clin Plast Surg 30(4):573–579
33. Pellegrini G, Ranno R, Stracuzzi G, Bondanza S, Guerra L, Zambruno G, Micali G, De Luca M (1999) The control of epidermal stem cells (holoclones) in the treatment of massive full-thickness burns with autologous keratinocytes cultured on fibrin. Transplantation 68(6):868–879
34. Khachemoune A, Bello YM, Phillips TJ (2002) Factors that influence healing in chronic venous ulcers treated with cryopreserved human epidermal cultures. Dermatol Surg 28(3):274–280
35. Alvarez-Diaz C, Cuenca-Pardo J, Sosa-Serrano A, Juarez-Aguilar E, Marsch-Moreno M, Kuri-Harcuch W (2000) Controlled clinical study of deep partial-thickness burns treated with frozen cultured human allogeneic epidermal sheets. J Burn Care Rehabil 21(4):291–299
36. Bolivar-Flores YJ, Kuri-Harcuch W (1999) Frozen allogeneic human epidermal cultured sheets for the cure of complicated leg ulcers. Dermatol Surg 25(8):610–617
37. Ponec M (2002) Skin constructs for replacement of skin tissues for in vitro testing. Adv Drug Deliv Rev 54(Suppl 1):S19–S30
38. Groeber F, Holeiter M, Hampel M, Hinderer S, Schenke-Layland K (2011) Skin tissue engineering – in vivo and in vitro applications. Adv Drug Deliv Rev 63(4–5):352–366
39. Wainwright DJ (1995) Use of an acellular allograft dermal matrix (AlloDerm) in the management of full-thickness burns. Burns 21(4):243–248
40. Supp DM, Boyce ST (2005) Engineered skin substitutes: practices and potentials. Clin Dermatol 23(4):403–412
41. Kolokol'chikova EG, Budkevich LI, Bobrovnikov AE, Badikova AK, Tumanov VP (2001) Morphological changes in burn wounds after transplantation of allogenic fibroblasts. Bull Exp Biol Med 131(1):89–93
42. Tompkins RG, Burke JF (1990) Progress in burn treatment and the use of artificial skin. World J Surg 14(6):819–824
43. Burke JF, Yannas IV, Quinby WC Jr, Bondoc CC, Jung WK (1981) Successful use of a physiologically acceptable artificial skin in the treatment of extensive burn injury. Ann Surg 194(4):413–428
44. Yannas IV, Burke JF, Orgill DP, Skrabut EM (1982) Wound tissue can utilize a polymeric template to synthesize a functional extension of skin. Science 215(4529):174–176
45. Yannas IV, Burke JF, Warpehoski M, Stasikelis P, Skrabut EM, Orgill D, Giard DJ (1981) Prompt, long-term functional replacement of skin. Trans Am Soc Artif Intern Organs 27:19–23
46. Branski LK, Herndon DN, Pereira C, Mlcak RP, Celis MM, Lee JO, Sanford AP, Norbury WB, Zhang XJ, Jeschke MG (2007) Longitudinal assessment of Integra in primary burn management: a randomized pediatric clinical trial. Crit Care Med 35(11):2615–2623
47. Clayman MA, Clayman SM, Mozingo DW (2006) The use of collagen-glycosaminoglycan copolymer (Integra) for the repair of hypertrophic scars and keloids. J Burn Care Res 27(3):404–409
48. Junkins-Hopkins JM (2011) Biologic dressings. J Am Acad Dermatol 64(1):e5–e7
49. Zaulyanov L, Kirsner RS (2007) A review of a bi-layered living cell treatment (Apligraf) in the treatment of venous leg ulcers and diabetic foot ulcers. Clin Interv Aging 2(1):93–98

50. Falanga V, Margolis D, Alvarez O, Auletta M, Maggiacomo F, Altman M, Jensen J, Sabolinski M, Hardin-Young J (1998) Rapid healing of venous ulcers and lack of clinical rejection with an allogeneic cultured human skin equivalent. Human Skin Equivalent Investigators Group. Arch Dermatol 134(3):293–300

51. Gohari S, Gambla C, Healey M, Spaulding G, Gordon KB, Swan J, Cook B, West DP, Lapiere JC (2002) Evaluation of tissue-engineered skin (human skin substitute) and secondary intention healing in the treatment of full thickness wounds after Mohs micrographic or excisional surgery. Dermatol Surg 28(12):1107–1114; discussion 1114

52. Eisenberg M, Llewelyn D (1998) Surgical management of hands in children with recessive dystrophic epidermolysis bullosa: use of allogeneic composite cultured skin grafts. Br J Plast Surg 51(8):608–613

53. Amado LC, Saliaris AP, Schuleri KH, St John M, Xie JS, Cattaneo S, Durand DJ, Fitton T, Kuang JQ, Stewart G et al (2005) Cardiac repair with intramyocardial injection of allogeneic mesenchymal stem cells after myocardial infarction. Proc Natl Acad Sci U S A 102(32): 11474–11479

54. Francois S, Mouiseddine M, Mathieu N, Semont A, Monti P, Dudoignon N, Sache A, Boutarfa A, Thierry D, Gourmelon P et al (2007) Human mesenchymal stem cells favour healing of the cutaneous radiation syndrome in a xenogenic transplant model. Ann Hematol 86(1):1–8

55. Badiavas EV, Falanga V (2003) Treatment of chronic wounds with bone marrow-derived cells. Arch Dermatol 139(4):510–516

56. Falanga V, Saap LJ, Ozonoff A (2006) Wound bed score and its correlation with healing of chronic wounds. Dermatol Ther 19(6):383–390

57. Altman AM, Matthias N, Yan Y, Song YH, Bai X, Chiu ES, Slakey DP, Alt EU (2008) Dermal matrix as a carrier for in vivo delivery of human adipose-derived stem cells. Biomaterials 29(10):1431–1442

58. Wu Y, Chen L, Scott PG, Tredget EE (2007) Mesenchymal stem cells enhance wound healing through differentiation and angiogenesis. Stem Cells 25(10):2648–2659

59. Kim WS, Park BS, Sung JH, Yang JM, Park SB, Kwak SJ, Park JS (2007) Wound healing effect of adipose-derived stem cells: a critical role of secretory factors on human dermal fibroblasts. J Dermatol Sci 48(1):15–24

60. Navsaria HA, Ojeh NO, Moiemen N, Griffiths MA, Frame JD (2004) Reepithelialization of a full-thickness burn from stem cells of hair follicles micrografted into a tissue-engineered dermal template (Integra). Plast Reconstr Surg 113(3):978–981

61. Inokuma D, Abe R, Fujita Y, Sasaki M, Shibaki A, Nakamura H, McMillan JR, Shimizu T, Shimizu H (2006) CTACK/CCL27 accelerates skin regeneration via accumulation of bone marrow-derived keratinocytes. Stem Cells 24(12):2810–2816

62. Sasaki M, Abe R, Fujita Y, Ando S, Inokuma D, Shimizu H (2008) Mesenchymal stem cells are recruited into wounded skin and contribute to wound repair by transdifferentiation into multiple skin cell type. J Immunol 180(4):2581–2587

63. Chambers SM, Goodell MA (2007) Hematopoietic stem cell aging: wrinkles in stem cell potential. Stem Cell Rev 3(3):201–211

64. Van Zant G, Liang Y (2003) The role of stem cells in aging. Exp Hematol 31(8):659–672

65. Schatteman GC, Ma N (2006) Old bone marrow cells inhibit skin wound vascularization. Stem Cells 24(3):717–721

Infections in Burns

4

Shahriar Shahrokhi

4.1 Burn Wound Infections

4.1.1 Diagnosis and Treatment of Burn Wound Infections

4.1.1.1 Introduction

Infections remain a leading cause of death in burn patients. This is as a result of loss of the environmental barrier function of the skin predisposing these patients to microbial colonization leading to invasion. Therefore, reconstitution of the environmental barrier by debriding the devitalized tissue and wound closure with application of allograft versus autograft is of optimal importance.

Given that infections are a common complication of the thermally injured patient, early diagnosis and treatment are of paramount importance. The pathophysiological progression of burn wound infection runs the spectrum from bacterial wound colonization to infection to invasive wound infection. The characteristics of each are as follows:

- *Bacterial colonization*
  - Bacterial levels $<10^5$
  - Does not necessarily prevent wound healing
- *Bacterial infection*
  - Bacterial levels $>10^5$
  - Can result in impaired wound healing and graft failure
  - Can lead to systemic infection
- *Invasive wound infection*
  - Clinically can have separation of the eschar from wound bed
  - Appearance of focal dark brown, black, or violaceous discoloration of the wound [1]

S. Shahrokhi, M.D., FRCSC
Division of Plastic and Reconstructive Surgery,
Ross Tilley Burn Centre, Sunnybrook Health Sciences Centre,
Bayview Ave 2075, Suite D716, Toronto, ON M4N 3M5, Canada
e-mail: shar.shahrokhi@sunnybrook.ca

M.G. Jeschke et al. (eds.), *Burn Care and Treatment*,
DOI 10.1007/978-3-7091-1133-8_4, © Springer-Verlag Wien 2013

Table 4.1 Common pathogens of burn wound infection

Organism	Common species
Gram-positive bacteria	*Staph* and *Strep* species
Gram-negative bacteria	*Pseudomonas aeruginosa, Acinetobacter baumannii, E. coli, Klebsiella pneumoniae, Enterobacter cloacae*
Yeast	*Candida sp.*
Fungi	*Aspergillus, Penicillium, Rhizopus, Mucor, Rhizomucor, Fusarium,* and *Curvularia*—have greater invasive potential
Virus	HSV, CMV
Multiresistant bacteria	MRSA, VRE, MDR *Pseudomonal* and *Acinetobacter* species

- Presence of pyocyanin (green pigment) in subcutaneous fat
- Erythema, edema, pain, and warmth of the surrounding skin
- Associated with signs of systemic infection/sepsis and positive blood cultures

Of note there are particular clinical signs unique to fungal and viral infections. An unexpected and rapid separation of the eschar is characteristic of fungal infection [2], while vesicular lesions caused by HSV-1 can be found in healed or healing burn wounds [3].

4.1.2 Common Pathogens and Diagnosis

In general the organisms causing burn wound infection/invasion have a chronological appearance. Initially, Gram-positive organisms are commonplace, while Gram-negative organisms become predominant after 5 days post-burn injury. Yeast and fungal colonization/infection follow, and finally multiresistant organisms appear typically as result of broad-spectrum antibiotics or inadequate burn excision or patient response to therapy [4].

As part of infection surveillance of burn patients, clinicians need to pay close attention to clinical signs of wound infection and rapidly confirm their diagnosis. There is some controversy as to the exact method of diagnosis, with some advocating for quantitative cultures—with $>10^5$ organisms per gram tissue being diagnostic of invasive infection [5]—and others arguing for histological examination as the only reliable method of determining invasive infection [6–9] since quantitative cultures are only positive in 50 % of histological invasive wound infections [9]. The most common pathogens of burn wound invasion are MSSA, MRSA, and *Pseudomonas aeruginosa* species (Table 4.1).

In order to provide the thermally injured patient with adequate treatment, it is important to have knowledge of each institution's bacterial flora as they vary with geography and over time [10, 11].

Fungal infections have increased in frequency with the use of topical agents, and the incidence of mycotic invasions has doubled. Even though the burn wound is the

Table 4.2 Topical agents and the antimicrobial activity

Agent	Affective against
Silver sulfadiazine	Gram-positives, gram-negatives, yeast
Mafenide acetate (5 %)	Gram-positives, gram-negatives
Silver nitrate (0.5 %)	Gram-positives, gram-negatives, yeast, fungi
Acetic acid (0.5 %, 2 %)	Gram-positives, gram-negatives, pseudomonas at higher concentration
Dakin's solution (0.25 % or 0.5 % sodium hypochlorite)	Gram-positives, gram-negatives, yeast, fungi
Acticoat	Gram-positives, gram-negatives, yeast, fungi, MRSA, VRE

most commonly infected site, there is an increasing trend toward systemic and organ-specific fungal infections [12].

The diagnosis of fungal infection is complicated by delay in their identification as cultures typically require 7–14 days [13], and their clinical presentation is similar to low-grade bacterial infections. Diagnosis can be aided by arterial blood samples as well retinal examination.

4.1.3 Clinical Management

Early excision and wound coverage is the mainstay of modern burn care and best method of minimizing burn wound infection. Any delay in the surgical treatment of burn wounds leads to increased bacterial loads, and any wound with bacterial counts exceeding 10^5 organisms per gram of tissue can develop burn wound sepsis even after burn wound excision [9].

The treatment of burn wound infections involves both local and systemic therapy.

4.1.3.1 Local
- Early excision of burn eschar (for un-excised burns)
- Aggressive excision of necrotic/infected tissue
- Topical agents (Table 4.2) to minimize bacterial colonization [14]

The use of any particular topical agent should be based on suspected organism in the wound but is at times guided by the availability of the agent on hospital formulary. These are not substitute for aggressive surgical management of wound infections.

4.1.3.2 Systemic
- Use of antibiotics and antifungals should be reserved for patients demonstrating systemic signs of sepsis (see ABA criteria for definition of sepsis (Box 4.1)).
- Use of systemic prophylaxis can reduce the rate of surgical wound infections but can increase bacterial antimicrobial resistance [15].
- The choice of antimicrobials needs to be based on each institution's antibiogram and tailored specifically to the organism (Table 4.3), i.e., narrow the coverage as soon as sensitivities become available.

Table 4.3 Ross Tilley Burn Centre guidelines for empiric antibiotic therapy

Early phase (<5 days)

The most common pathogens (from any source) in the *early* phase of a patient's admission are:

Gram-positive

Staphylococcus aureus (~90 % susceptible to cloxacillin)

Gram-negatives (95 % susceptibility to ceftriaxone)

H. influenza

E. coli

Klebsiella spp.

Based on this data, septic patients admitted within the past 5 days should be started on an empiric regimen of:

Ceftriaxone 1 g IV q24 h

+/− Cloxacilliin 1–2 g IV q4–6 h (renal dosing required)

Penicillin allergy

Levofloxacin 750 mg IV/PO q24 h

Late phase (>5 days)

The most common pathogens (from any source) in the *late* phase of a patient's admission are:

Gram-positive

Staphylococcus aureus (only ~60 % susceptible to cloxacillin)

Gram-negative (generally more predominant in the late phase)

Pseudomonas aeruginosa (>80 % susceptible to piperacillin/tazobactam)

Based on this data, septic patients admitted 5 days or more should be started on an empiric regimen of:

Piperacillin/tazobactam 4.5 g IV q6 h (renal dosing required)

+ Vancomycin 1 g IV q12 h (with pre- and post-levels around the third dose)

Or

Meropenem 500 mg IV q6 h (renal dosing required)

- Yeast species (*Candida*) are typically sensitive to fluconazole, while fungal infections would most likely require treatment with amphotericin or caspofungin (the use is for systemic infection, as wound infections require surgical debridement).
- Viral infections (typically HSV) require treatment with acyclovir.

> **Box 4.1 ABA Criteria for Definition of Sepsis [16]**
> Includes at least three of the following:
> Temperature >39° or <36.5 °C
> Progressive tachycardia
> - Adults >110 bpm
> - Children >2 SD above age-specific norms (85 % age-adjusted max heart rate)

Progressive tachypnea
- Adults >25 bpm not ventilated. Minute ventilation >12 L/min ventilated
- Children >2 SD above age-specific norms (85 % age-adjusted max respiratory rate)

Thrombocytopenia (will not apply until 3 days after initial resuscitation)
- Adults <100,000/mcl
- Children >2 SD below age-specific norms

Hyperglycemia (in the absence of preexisting diabetes mellitus)
- Untreated plasma glucose >200 mg/dL or equivalent mM/L
- Insulin resistance—examples include:
  - >7 units of insulin/h intravenous drip (adults)
  - Significant resistance to insulin (>25 % increase in insulin requirements over 24 h)

Inability to continue enteral feedings >24 h
- Abdominal distension
- Enteral feeding intolerance (residual >150 mL/h in children or two times feeding rate in adults)
- Uncontrollable diarrhea (>2,500 mL/day for adults or >400 mL/day in children)

In addition, it is *required* that a documented infection (defined below) is identified:
- Culture-positive infection
- Pathologic tissue source identified
- Clinical response to antimicrobials

Infections of burn wounds are typically found in patients with burns exceeding 20 % TBSA and most commonly in the lower extremities [17]. However, there are no specific organisms associated with the site of infection [17]. Moreover, these infections can have dire consequences:
- Conversion of superficial to deeper burn wounds
- Systemic infection and sepsis
- Graft loss requiring further surgery for regrafting
- Increased hospital length of stay
- Conversion of donor sites requiring surgical debridement and grafting
- Increased mortality, more so with yeast and fungal infection

4.1.4 Conclusion

Burn wound infection is an all too common complication of the thermally injured patient. These infections tend to have a chronological appearance and depend on burn size, depth, length of hospital stay, and geographical location. The common organisms remain *Staphylococcus* and *Pseudomonas*; however, more resistant strains are becoming prevalent. The clinician needs to be vigilant with surveillance of burn wounds and institute aggressive treatment of wound infection once clinical signs appear before systemic illness sets in. It is of utmost importance to have ongoing assessment of the unique flora of each institution in order to better utilize systemic therapy.

4.2   Ventilator-Associated Pneumonia

Ventilator-associated pneumonia (VAP) as defined by CDC (Center for Diseases Control) is an infection that occurs in a mechanically ventilated patient with an endotracheal or tracheostomy tube (traditionally >48 h after hospital admission) [18, 19]. The diagnosis of VAP in the thermally injured patient can be challenging, as fever, leukocytosis, tachycardia, and tachypnea can be present in these patients without infection. The sources of bacteria are typically the oropharynx and upper gastrointestinal tract [20–24]. The organisms also have a temporal pattern, community-acquired organisms (*Streptococcus pneumoniae and Haemophilus influenza*) are dominant in the early-phase VAP and Gram-negative and multiresistant organisms (i.e., MRSA) are the common pathogens in late-stage VAP.

Regardless of the organisms, early antimicrobial treatment guided toward the likely organism based on the onset of VAP (early vs. late) is beneficial in the overall outcome of the patients [25–30]. These broad-spectrum antimicrobials would need to be de-escalated as culture and sensitivities become available [31–33].

As VAP is an increasing common complication with significant consequences, VAP prevention strategies need to be implemented and ABA guidelines (Box 4.2) utilized to improve overall patient outcome.

Box 4.2 American Burn Association Practice Guidelines for Prevention, Diagnosis, and Treatment of Ventilator-Associated Pneumonia (VAP) in Burn Patients [34]

- Mechanically ventilated burn patients are at high risk for developing VAP, with the presence of inhalation injury as a unique risk factor in this patient group.
- VAP prevention strategies should be used in mechanically ventilated burn patients.
- Clinical diagnosis of VAP can be challenging in mechanically ventilated burn patients where systemic inflammation and acute lung injury are prevalent. Therefore, a quantitative strategy, when available, is the preferable method to confirm the diagnosis of VAP.
- An 8-day course of targeted antibiotic therapy is generally sufficient to treat VAP; however, resistant *Staphylococcus aureus* and Gram-negative bacilli may require longer treatment duration.

4.3 Central Line-Associated Infections

Central catheters inserted into veins and arteries are common practice in the management of the critically ill thermally injured patient and can be associated with infection rates from 1.5 to 20 % [35–37]. The introduction of central line insertion bundles by CDC has dramatically reduced these infections [38, 39]. These measures include:

- Hand washing
- Full-barrier precautions during line insertion
- Cleaning the skin with chlorhexidine
- Avoiding the femoral site if possible
- Removing unnecessary catheters

In burn patients some unique features complicate the use of the central catheters. Typically there are associated burn wounds in close proximity, and it has been shown that catheters within 25 cm^2 of an open wound are at an increased risk of colonization and infection [40]. Other risk factors associated with increased rate of infection are [41]:

- Age (extremes of age have more infection)
- Sex (female)
- %TBSA burned
- % full-thickness burns
- Presence of smoke inhalation
- Type of burn (flame)
- Number of surgical procedures performed
- Larger number of CVCs
- Longer insertion of the catheter
- Wound burn infection or colonization
- Insertion of the venous catheter in emergency situation
- Longer stay in hospital
- More operations
- Insertion site near the burns wound

The diagnosis of catheter-related infection (CRI) is based on clinical and microbiological criteria (see Table 4.4). Following the diagnosis of CRI prompt treatment is essential as delay in catheter removal or in the start of appropriate antimicrobial therapy can result in increased morbidity and mortality [43].

Currently there is no clear evidence that routine exchange of lines decreases the rate of catheter-related blood stream infections (CRBSI) [44]; however, all catheters need to be removed once a CRBSI is diagnosed or once they are no longer needed.

As with all severe infections empiric antimicrobial treatment should be initiated immediately and should take into account the severity of the illness, the site of catheter insertion, and the institutions' antibiogram [45]. These broad-spectrum antimicrobials need to be de-escalated after identification and susceptibility testing of the microorganism.

Table 4.4 Catheter-related infection [42]

Type of infection	Criteria
Catheter colonization	A significant growth of a microorganism from the catheter tip, subcutaneous segment, or catheter hub in the absence of clinical signs of infection
Exit-site infection	Microbiologically documented exudates at catheter exit site yield a microorganism with or without concomitant bloodstream infection.
	Clinically documented erythema or induration within 2 cm of the catheter exit site in the absence of associated bloodstream infection and without concomitant purulence
Positive blood culture	Microorganism, potentially pathogenic, cultured from one or more blood culture
Bloodstream infection	Positive blood culture with a clinical sepsis (see below)
Clinical sepsis	Requires one of the following with no other recognized cause: fever (>38 °C), hypotension (SBP <90 mmHg), oliguria, paired quantitative blood cultures with a >5:1 ratio catheter versus peripheral, differential time to positivity (blood culture obtained from a CVC is positive at least 2 h earlier than a peripheral blood culture)

4.4   Guidelines for Sepsis Resuscitation

As described in the previous segments of this chapter, infections in the thermally injured patient have dire consequences. Sepsis occurs at a rate of 8–42.5 % in burn patients with a mortality of 28–65 % [46]. Much research has been conducted in the optimal management of the septic patient. The following Table 4.5 summarizes the guidelines as recommended by the surviving sepsis campaign committee [47]. Only the strong recommendations with high level of evidence are included. This is to be used as a tool to guide the delivery of optimal clinical care for patients with sepsis and septic shock. The ABA criteria for definition of sepsis (see Box 4.1) in the burn patients have been established. However, Mann-Salinas and colleagues have challenged the predictive ability of ABA criteria demonstrating that their multivariable model (heart rate >130, MAP <60 mmHg, base deficit <−6 mEq/L, temperature <36 °C, use of vasoactive medications, and glucose >150 mg/dL) is capable of outperforming the ABA model [48].

Table 4.5 Guidelines for management of sepsis and septic shock [47][a]

Initial resuscitation (first 6 h)	Begin resuscitation immediately in patients with hypotension or elevated serum lactate >4 mmol/L; do not delay pending ICU admission
	Resuscitation goals:
	CVP 8–12 mmHg
	Mean arterial pressure ≥65 mmHg
	Urine output ≥0.5 mL/kg/h
	Central venous (superior vena cava) oxygen saturation ≥70 % or mixed venous ≥65 %
Diagnosis	Obtain appropriate cultures before starting antibiotics provided this does not significantly delay antimicrobial administration
	Obtain two or more BCs
	One or more BCs should be percutaneous
	One BC from each vascular access device in place >48 h
	Culture other sites as clinically indicated
	Perform imaging studies promptly to confirm and sample any source of infection, if safe to do so
Antibiotic therapy	Begin intravenous antibiotics as early as possible and always within the first hour of recognizing severe sepsis and septic shock
	Broad-spectrum: one or more agents active against likely bacterial/fungal pathogens and with good penetration into presumed source
	Reassess antimicrobial regimen daily to optimize efficacy, prevent resistance, avoid toxicity, and minimize costs
	Consider combination therapy in Pseudomonas infections
	Consider combination empiric therapy in neutropenic patients
	Combination therapy ≤3–5 days and de-escalation following susceptibilities
	Duration of therapy typically limited to 7–10 days; longer if response is slow or there are undrainable foci of infection or immunologic deficiencies
	Stop antimicrobial therapy if cause is found to be noninfectious
Source identification and control	A specific anatomic site of infection should be established as rapidly as possible and within first 6 h of presentation
	Formally evaluate patient for a focus of infection amenable to source control measures (e.g., abscess drainage, tissue debridement)
	Implement source control measures as soon as possible following successful initial resuscitation (exception: infected pancreatic necrosis, where surgical intervention is best delayed)
	Choose source control measure with maximum efficacy and minimal physiologic upset. Remove intravascular access devices if potentially infected

(continued)

Table 4.5 (continued)

Fluid therapy	Fluid-resuscitate using crystalloids or colloids
	Target a CVP of ≥8 mmHg (≥12 mmHg if mechanically ventilated)
	Use a fluid challenge technique while associated with a hemodynamic improvement
	Give fluid challenges of 1,000 mL of crystalloids or 300–500 mL of colloids over 30 min. More rapid and larger volumes may be required in sepsis-induced tissue hypoperfusion
	Rate of fluid administration should be reduced if cardiac filling pressures increase without concurrent hemodynamic improvement
Vasopressors	Maintain MAP ≥65 mmHg
	Norepinephrine and dopamine centrally administered are the initial vasopressors of choice
	Do not use low-dose dopamine for renal protection
	In patients requiring vasopressors, insert an arterial catheter as soon as practical
Inotropic therapy	Use dobutamine in patients with myocardial dysfunction as supported by elevated cardiac filling pressures and low cardiac output
	Do not increase cardiac index to predetermined supernormal levels
Steroids	Do not use corticosteroids to treat sepsis in the absence of shock unless the patient's endocrine or corticosteroid history warrants it
Recombinant human activated protein C	Adult patients with severe sepsis and low risk of death (typically, APACHE II <20 or one organ failure) should not receive rhAPC
Blood product administration	Give red blood cells when hemoglobin decreases to <7.0 g/dL (<70 g/L) to target hemoglobin of 7.0–9.0 g/dL in adults. A higher hemoglobin level may be required in special circumstances (e.g., myocardial ischemia, severe hypoxemia, acute hemorrhage, cyanotic heart disease, or lactic acidosis)
	Do not use antithrombin therapy
Mechanical ventilation of sepsis-induced ALI/ARDS	Target a tidal volume of 6 mL/kg (predicted) body weight in patients with ALI/ARDS
	Target an initial upper limit plateau pressure ≤30 cm H_2O. Consider chest wall compliance when assessing plateau pressure
	Allow $PaCO_2$ to increase above normal, if needed, to minimize plateau pressures and tidal volumes
	Set PEEP to avoid extensive lung collapse at end expiration
	Maintain mechanically ventilated patients in a semi-recumbent position (head of the bed raised to 45°) unless contraindicated
	Use a weaning protocol and an SBT regularly to evaluate the potential for discontinuing mechanical ventilation
	SBT options include a low level of pressure support with continuous positive airway pressure 5 cm H_2O or a T piece
	Do not use a pulmonary artery catheter for the routine monitoring of patients with ALI/ARDS
	Use a conservative fluid strategy for patients with established ALI who do not have evidence of tissue hypoperfusion

Sedation, analgesia, and neuromuscular blockade in sepsis	Use sedation protocols with a sedation goal for critically ill mechanically ventilated patients
	Use either intermittent bolus sedation or continuous infusion sedation to predetermined end points (sedation scales), with daily interruption/lightening to produce awakening
	Avoid neuromuscular blockers where possible. Monitor depth of block with train-of-four when using continuous infusions
Glucose control	Use intravenous insulin to control hyperglycemia in patients with severe sepsis following stabilization in the ICU
	Aim to keep blood glucose <150 mg/dL (8.3 mmol/L) using a validated protocol for insulin dose adjustment
	Provide a glucose calorie source and monitor blood glucose values every 1–2 h (4 h when stable) in patients receiving intravenous insulin
	Interpret with caution low glucose levels obtained with point of care testing, as these techniques may overestimate arterial blood or plasma glucose values
Bicarbonate therapy	Do not use bicarbonate therapy for the purpose of improving hemodynamics or reducing vasopressor requirements when treating hypoperfusion-induced lactic acidemia with pH ≥7.15
DVT prophylaxis	Use a mechanical prophylactic device, such as compression stockings or an intermittent compression device, when heparin is contraindicated
	Use either low-dose UFH or LMWH, unless contraindicated
Stress ulcer prophylaxis	Provide stress ulcer prophylaxis using H2 blocker or proton pump inhibitor
Consideration for limitation of support	Discuss advance care planning with patients and families. Describe likely outcomes and set realistic expectations

[a]Adapted from Dellinger et al. [47]

References

1. Pruitt BA, Lindberg RB, McManus WF, Mason AD (1983) Current approach to prevention and treatment of Pseudomonas aeruginosa infections in burned patients. Rev Infect Dis 5(Suppl 5):S889–S897
2. Pruitt BA (1984) The diagnosis and treatment of infection in the burn patient. Burns Incl Therm Inj 11(2):79–91
3. Foley FD, Greenawald KA, Nash G, Pruitt BA (1970) Herpesvirus infection in burned patients. N Engl J Med 282(12):652–656
4. Church D, Elsayed S, Reid O, Winston B, Lindsay R (2006) Burn wound infections. Mol Biol Rep 19:403–434
5. Heggers JP, Robson MC (eds) (1991) Quantitative bacteriology: its role in the armamentarium of the surgeon, 1st edn. CRC Press, Boca Raton
6. McManus AT, Kim SH, McManus WF, Mason AD, Pruitt BA (1987) Comparison of quantitative microbiology and histopathology in divided burn-wound biopsy specimens. Arch Surg 122(1):74–76
7. Pruitt BA, McManus AT (1992) The changing epidemiology of infections in burn patients. World J Surg 16(1):57–67

8. Pruitt BA, McManus AT, Kim SH, Goodwin CW (1998) Burn wound infections: current status. World J Surg 22(2):135–145
9. Barret JP, Herndon DN (2003) Effects of burn wound excision on bacterial colonization and invasion. Plast Reconstr Surg 111(2):744–750
10. Guggenheim M, Zbinden R, Handschin AE, Gohritz A, Altintas MA, Giovanoli P (2009) Changes in bacterial isolates from burn wounds and their antibiograms: a 20-year study (1986–2005). Burns 35(4):553–560
11. Rezaei E, Safari H, Naderinasab M, Aliakbarian H (2011) Common pathogens in burn wound and changes in their drug sensitivity. Burns 37(5):805–807
12. Sheridan RL (2005) Sepsis in pediatric burn patients. Pediatr Crit Care Med 6(3 Suppl): S112–S119
13. Becker WK, Cioffi WG Jr, McManus AT, Kim SH, McManus WF, Mason AD et al (1991) Fungal burn wound infection. A 10-year experience. Arch Surg 126(1):44–48
14. Greenhalgh DG (2009) Topical antimicrobial agents for burn wounds. Clin Plast Surg 36(4):597–606
15. Avni T, Levcovich A, Ad-El DD, Leibovici L, Paul M (2010) Prophylactic antibiotics for burns patients: systematic review and meta-analysis. BMJ 340:c241
16. Greenhalgh DG, The American Burn Association Consensus Conference on Burn Sepsis and Infection Group et al (2007) American burn association consensus conference to define sepsis and infection in burns. J Burn Care Res 28(6):776–790
17. Posluszny JA Jr, Conrad P, Halerz M, Shankar R, Gamelli RL (2011) Surgical burn wound infections and their clinical implications. J Burn Care Res 32:324–333
18. Centers for Disease Control and Prevention (2004) Guidelines for preventing health-care–associated pneumonia, 2003: recommendations of CDC and the Healthcare Infection Control Practices Advisory Committee. MMWR Recomm Rep 53:1–36
19. Centers for Disease Control and Prevention (2008) The National Healthcare Safety Network (NHSN) manual: patient safety component protocol 2007. Available from: http://www.cdc.gov/ncidod/dhqp/pdf/nhsn/NHSN_Manual_PatientSafetyProtocol_CURRENT.pdf; Internet; Accessed 14 Dec 2008
20. Cook D, Walter S, Cook R et al (1998) Incidence of and risk factors for ventilator-associated pneumonia in critically ill patients. Ann Intern Med 129:433–440
21. Bahrani-Mougeot F, Paster B, Coleman S et al (2007) Molecular analysis of oral and respiratory bacterial species associated with ventilator-associated pneumonia. J Clin Microbiol 45:1588–1593
22. DeRiso AJ II, Ladowski JS, Dillon TA, Justice JW, Peterson AC (1996) Chlorhexidine gluconate 0.12 % oral rinse reduces the incidence of total nosocomial respiratory infection and non-prophylactic systemic antibiotic use in patients undergoing heart surgery. Chest 109:1556–1561
23. Seguin P, Tanguy M, Laviolle B, Tirel O, Mallédant Y (2006) Effect of oropharyngeal decontamination by povidone-iodine on ventilator-associated pneumonia in patients with head trauma. Crit Care Med 34:1514–1519
24. Bonten MJ, Gaillard CA, de Leeuw PW, Stobberingh EE (1997) Role of colonization of the upper intestinal tract in the pathogenesis of ventilator-associated pneumonia. Clin Infect Dis 24:309–319
25. Iregui M, Ward S, Sherman G, Fraser VJ, Kollef MH (2002) Clinical importance of delays in the initiation of appropriate antibiotic treatment for ventilator-associated pneumonia. Chest 122:262–268
26. Garnacho-Montero J, Garcia-Garmendia JL, Barrero-Almodovar A et al (2003) Impact of the outcome of adequate empirical antibiotherapy in patients admitted to the ICU for sepsis. Crit Care Med 31:2742–2751
27. Leone M, Burgoin A, Cambon S, Dubuc M, Albanèse J, Martin C (2003) Empirical antimicrobial therapy of septic shock patients: adequacy and impact on the outcome. Crit Care Med 31:462–467
28. Luna CM, Vujacich P, Niederman MS et al (1997) Impact of BAL data on the therapy and outcome of ventilator-associated pneumonia. Chest 111:676–685

29. Rello J, Gallego M, Mariscal D, Soñora R, Valles J (1997) The value of routine microbial investigation in ventilator-associated pneumonia. Am J Respir Crit Care Med 156:196–200

30. Dupont H, Mentec H, Sollet JP, Bleichner G (2001) Impact of appropriateness of initial antibiotic therapy on the outcome of ventilator-associated pneumonia. Intensive Care Med 27: 355–362

31. Alvarez-Lerma F (1996) Modification of empiric antibiotic treatment in patients with pneumonia acquired in the intensive care unit. ICU-acquired Pneumonia Study Group. Intensive Care Med 22:387–394

32. Ibrahim EH, Ward S, Sherman G, Schaiff R, Fraser VJ, Kollef MH (2001) Experience with a clinical guideline for the treatment of ventilator-associated pneumonia. Crit Care Med 29:1109–1115

33. Namias N, Samiian L, Nino D et al (2000) Incidence and susceptibility of pathogenic bacteria vary between intensive care units within a single hospital: implications for empiric antibiotic strategies. J Trauma 49:638–645

34. Mosier MJ, Pham TN (2009) American burn association practice guidelines for prevention, diagnosis, and treatment of ventilator-associated pneumonia (VAP) in burn patients. J Burn Care Res 30:910–928

35. Franceschi D, Gerding R, Phillips G, Fratianne R (1989) Risk factors associated with intravascular catheter infections in burned patients: a prospective, randomized study. J Trauma 29:811–816

36. Goldestein A, Weber J, Sheridan R (1997) Femoral venous access is safe in burned children, an analysis of 224 catheters. J Pediatr 130:442–446

37. Lesseva M (1998) Central venous catheter-related bacteremia in burn patients. Scand J Infect Dis 30:585–589

38. Berenholtz SM, Pronovost PJ, Lipsett PA et al (2004) Eliminating catheter-related bloodstream infections in the intensive care unit. Crit Care Med 32:2014–2020

39. Pronovost P, Needham D, Berenholtz S et al (2006) An intervention to decrease catheter-related bloodstream infections in the ICU. N Engl J Med 355:2725–2732

40. Ramos GE, Bolgiani AN, Patiño O, Prezzavento GE, Guastavino P, Durlach R, Fernandez Canigia LB, Fortunato Benaim F (2002) Catheter infection risk related to the distance between insertion site and burned area. J Burn Care Rehabil 23:266–271

41. Echevarria-Guanilo ME, Ciofi-Silva CL, Canini SR, Farina JA, Rossi LA (2009) Preventing infections due to intravascular catheters in burn victims. Expert Rev Anti Infect Ther 7(9):1081–1086

42. Pagani JL, Eggimann P (2008) Management of catheter-related infection. Expert Rev Anti Infect Ther 6(1):31–37

43. Warren DK, Quadir WW, Hollenbeak CS, Elward AM, Cox MJ, Fraser VJ (2006) Attributable cost of catheter-associated bloodstream infections among intensive care patients in a nonteaching hospital. Crit Care Med 34(8):2084–2089

44. O'Mara MS, Reed NL, Palmieri TL, Greenhalgh DG (2007) Central venous catheter infections in burn patients with scheduled catheter exchange and replacement. J Surg Res 142(2): 341–350

45. Lorente L, Jimenez A, Iribarren JL, Jimenez JJ, Martin MM, Mora ML (2006) The microorganism responsible for central venous catheter related bloodstream infection depends on catheter site. Intensive Care Med 32(9):1449–1450

46. Mann EA, Baun MM, Meininger JC, Wade CE (2012) Comparison of mortality associated with sepsi in the burn, trauma, and general intensive care unit patient: a systematic review of the literature. Shock 37(1):4–16

47. Dellinger RP, International Surviving Sepsis Campaign Guidelines Committee et al (2008) Surviving sepsis campaign: international guidelines for management of severe sepsis and septic shock: 2008. Crit Care Med 36(1):296–327

48. Mann-Salinas EA, Baun MM, Meininger JC, Murray CK, Aden JK, Wolf SE, Wade CE (2013) Novel predictors of sepsis outperform the American burn association sepsis criteria in the burn intensive care unit patient. J Burn Care Res 34(1):31–43

Acute Burn Surgery

5

Lars-Peter Kamolz

5.1 Introduction

During the past decades, burn care has improved to the extent that persons with burns can frequently survive (Fig. 5.1). The trend in current burn care extends beyond the preservation of life; the ultimate goal is the return of burn victims, as full participants, back into their families and communities.

5.2 Burn Wound Evaluation

One of the major problems that face any burn surgeon is the decision on the nature of treatment (conservative treatment versus operative treatment). In the case of an operative procedure, a decision is needed on when and how to excise the burn wounds and to determine accurately the depth of the lesion and thereby the extent of tissue involvement.

5.3 Escharotomy/Fasciotomy

One of the most important indications for an immediate surgical intervention is the presence of a compartment syndrome. Circumferential burns have a high risk to develop compartment syndrome. Compartment syndrome can occur in circumferential upper and lower extremity burns, but escharotomy may be necessary also to relieve chest wall restriction in order to improve ventilation.

L.-P. Kamolz, MD, PhD, MSc
Division of Plastic, Aesthetic and Reconstructive Surgery,
Department of Surgery, Medical University of Graz,
Auenbruggerplatz 29, 8036 Graz, Austria
e-mail: lars.kamolz@medunigraz.at

M.G. Jeschke et al. (eds.), *Burn Care and Treatment*,
DOI 10.1007/978-3-7091-1133-8_5, © Springer-Verlag Wien 2013

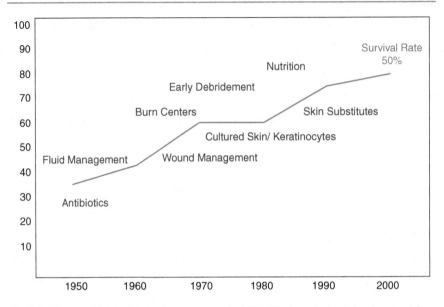

Fig. 5.1 Factors which had major impact on survival. The 50 % survival rate has increased from 35 % TBSA to 80 % TBSA within the past decades

5.4   Surgical Burn Wound Management

The main goal of surgical treatment is the replacement of necrotic tissue. One of the main problems encountered in extensively burned patients >60 % total body surface area (TBSA) is the scarcity of harvesting areas for autologous skin grafts.

Superficial dermal burns will heal without operation within 2–3 weeks, but deep dermal and full-thickness burn will require operation. It is widely accepted that if skin does not regenerate within 3 weeks, morbidity and scarring will be severe, so the trend in the treatment of deep dermal and full-thickness burns leans toward very early excision and grafting in order to reduce the risk of infection, decrease scar formation, shorten hospital stay and thereby reduce costs.

Excision of as much of the necrotic tissue as possible should be carried out whenever a patient is hemodynamically stable and the risks of the operation would not increase the mortality that would be expected from the traditional treatment. In patients with associated injuries such as inhalation injury, patients of extreme age, or patients with cardiac problems, special surgical treatment is required in deciding when and how much to excise.

Sequential layered tangential excision to viable bleeding points, even to fat, while minimising the loss of viable tissue, is the generally accepted technique.

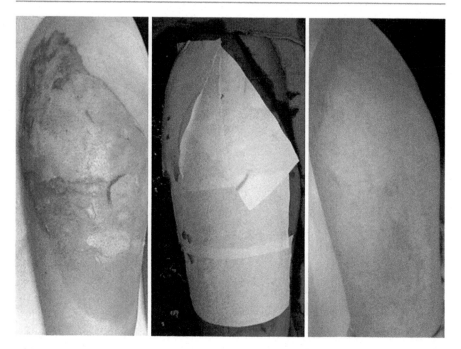

Fig. 5.2 Mixed dermal burn—tangential excision of the deeper parts and coverage with Suprathel®, late results

Excision of burn wounds to the fascia is reserved for large burns where the risks of massive blood loss and the possibility of skin slough from less vascularised grafts on fat may lead to higher mortality.

We start to excise all deep dermal and full-thickness burned areas within 72 h of injury. It has become apparent that early excision is better than late excision, because after 7 days the incidence of sepsis and graft failure increases:

In case of deep dermal injuries, after tangential excision the resulting defects can be covered with keratinocytes, autologous or allogeneic skin grafts or by use of synthetic materials like Suprathel® (Fig. 5.2).

In case of full-thickness burns, we dominantly use autografts to cover the wounds if there are sufficient available donor sites. In large burns we normally use expanded autografts (mesh or Meek).

Expansion rates of graft to wound area cover ranges from 1: 1 to 1: 9. Expansion rates higher than 1: 3 heal in a suboptimal manner leading to contractures and unstable scars. Therefore, we like to combine these large meshed autografts in combination with allografts (Fig. 5.3) or keratinocytes (sandwich technique), or we will use the Meek technique (Fig. 5.4). In functional important regions like hands and over joints, a combined reconstruction of skin by use of a dermal matrix (Integra®, Matriderm®), and split-thickness skin graft seems to be superior to skin grafts alone (Fig. 5.5).

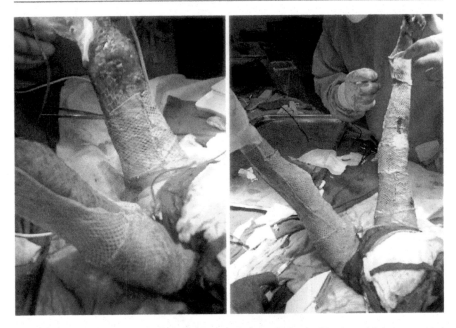

Fig. 5.3 "Sandwich technique": widely expanded autografts in combination with less expanded allografts

Fig. 5.4 Direct comparison of mesh and Meek grafted area

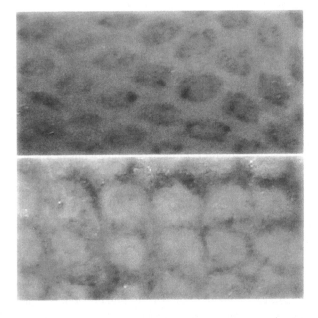

Donor sites for autografts in smaller burns, less than 40 % total body surface area, are seldom a problem unless the patient is at risk of surgical complication resulting from age, cardiopulmonary problems, or coagulopathy. Patients with greater burns have a lack of available donor sites. Therefore, we use cadaver skin

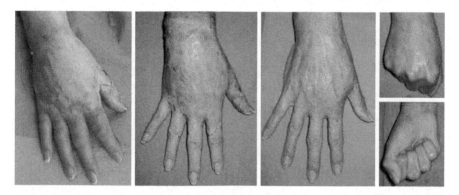

Fig. 5.5 Dermal to full-thickness burn: excision and combined grafting (Matriderm® and unmeshed skin graft); early and late results

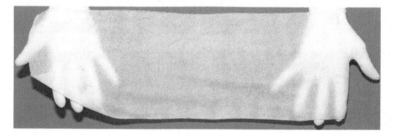

Fig. 5.6 Pigskin (EZ-Derm®) as a temporary coverage of full-thickness burns in case of a lack of donor sites for autologous skin grafting

(allografts) or xenografts (Fig. 5.6) as a temporary transplant and cover. These temporary transplants decrease the size of open wound until autografts become available as the partial-thickness burn area is healed or previously harvested donor sites heal.

This temporary covering helps to:
- Control wound infection
- Prevent wound contracture
- Relieve pain

Sometimes, due to the fact that burn wounds are often a combination of different burn depth, different techniques are combined in order to optimise burn wound closure concerning healing time and quality (Fig. 5.7).

5.5   Location-Specific Treatment

5.5.1   Face

Deep dermal burns will be debrided and covered with keratinocytes or by silver-containing dressings like Acticoat Flex®. Full-thickness burns will be excised and grafted with unmeshed skin grafts according to aesthetic units of the face.

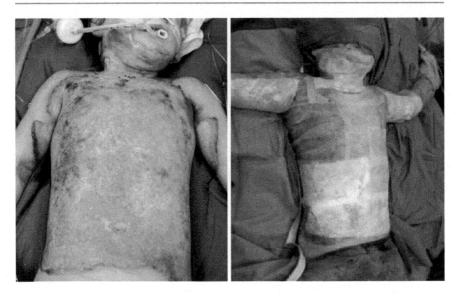

Fig. 5.7 Dermal to full-thickness burn. Tangential excision and grafting: deep dermal parts with Suprathel®, full-thickness parts with meshed skin grafts (1:2)

5.5.2 Hands

Deep dermal burns will be debrided and covered with keratinocytes, unmeshed skin grafts, or synthetic materials like Suprathel®. Full-thickness burns will be excised and grafted with unmeshed skin grafts, sometimes in combination with dermal substitutes.

5.6 Treatment Standards in Burns Larger Than Sixty Percent TBSA

Body region can be organised according to the probability of skin take rate and functional importance and ultimately determined for surgical priority (Figs. 5.8 and 5.9).

The aim of surgical strategy is to remove the necrotic tissue within 9 days after injury; in large burns the dorsal aspects of the lower extremities, dorsum, gluteal and dorsal femoral regions can be preferably preconditioned in a fluidised microsphere beads-bed, and the final debridement is normally not performed before days 10–14 after injury.

Excision and grafting sessions can be organised in a timeline scheme described in Fig. 5.9:

- In young and clinically stable adult burn patients, we aimed to remove necrotic tissue and provide cover for full-thickness burns in two operative sessions within the first 14 days after injury.

Definition	Body region
funtional & aesthetic importance	face hands feet
superior take-rate	thorax, abdomen upper limb lower limb
inferior take-rate	flanks of torso gluteal region dorsal aspect of thighs

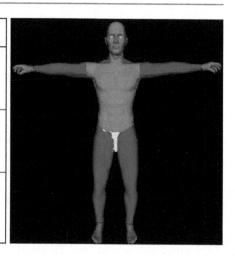

Fig. 5.8 Body region organisation based on the functional importance and take rate

Timeline	Body region	Preferred technique
Day 3-9	hands	unmeshed split-thickness skin grafts (STSG)
	thorax, abdomen upper extremity ventral lower extremity	Meek (1:6 or 1:9) Mesh (1:1.5 or 1:3)
Day 10-14	face	unmeshed STSG
	dorsum dorsal lower extremity gluteal regions dorsal aspect of thigh	Meek (1:6 or 1:9) Mesh (1:1.5 or 1:3)
> Day 14	residual defects	Mesh (1:1.5 or 1:3)

Fig. 5.9 Surgical timeline

- Individuals aged 65 years and above usually required more than two operative sessions within the first 14 days, because the area operated on per session had to be restrained and adapted to the patient's general condition.

Whenever possible, unmeshed split-thickness skin grafts (STSG) are used for face and hands; all other areas are covered with either Meek grafts (expansion ratio 1:6 or 1:9) or, if respective donor sites sufficient, with mesh grafts using an expansion ratio of 1:1.5 or 1:3. Expansion ratios exceeding 1:3 to achieve sufficient coverage for full-thickness burns are regarded as indication for using the Meek technique (1:6 or 1:9).

5.7   Temporary Coverage

If harvested STSG did not suffice for coverage of full-thickness areas (third degree), we prefer to use allogeneic STSG as temporary alternative. However, if allogeneic skin is not available, we use xenografts or a synthetic material (Epigard®) to temporarily cover debrided full-thickness areas.

Surgical priority is given to areas of functional and aesthetic importance and superior take rate. Body regions with inferior take rate are normally preconditioned.

5.8   Fluidised Microsphere Beads-Bed

Fluidised microsphere beads-beds can be used for wound preconditioning but also for postoperative wound care. This method allows the removal of moisture in order to keep wounds dry and to permit maintenance of constant temperature levels in areas in direct contact with the bed's superficial fabric. Only thin sterile covers are employed to shield dorsal burned areas while in these beds, and no extra ointments are applied. For wound coverage of freshly operated areas, we prefer to use fat gauzes and dry sterile compresses.

Patients with arising difficulties in respiratory management or temperature control while in fluidised microsphere beads-beds were temporarily transferred to standard intensive care beds.

5.9   Negative-Pressure Wound Therapy (Vacuum-Assisted Closure)

Negative-pressure wound therapy or vacuum-assisted closure (VAC®) can be used the local therapy in STSG receiver regions of inferior take and allowed for early mobilisation in functionally important zones.

5.9.1   Early Mobilisation

Early individual physiotherapy and ergotherapeutic splinting accomplishes the therapeutic strategy.

5.9.2   Nutrition and Anabolic Agents

Catabolism as a response to thermal trauma can only be modulated, not completely reversed. The burn wound consumes large quantities of energy during the healing process due to the large population of inflammatory cells and the production of collagen and matrix by fibroblasts. Therefore, adequate nutrition is of utmost importance for burn wound healing.

Bibliography

1. Amis BP, Klein MB (2012) Hand burns. In: Jeschke MG, Kamolz LP, Sjöberg F, Wolf SE (eds) Handbook of burns, vol 1, Acute burn care. Springer, Wien, pp 303–310
2. Branski LK, Dibildox M, Shahrokhi S, Jeschke MG (2012) Treatment of burns – established and novel technology. In: Jeschke MG, Kamolz LP, Sjöberg F, Wolf SE (eds) Handbook of burns, vol 1, Acute burn care. Springer, Wien, pp 311–324
3. Dziewulski P, Villapalos JL (2012) Acute management of facial burns. In: Jeschke MG, Kamolz LP, Sjöberg F, Wolf SE (eds) Handbook of burns, vol 1, Acute burn care. Springer, Wien, pp 291–302
4. Engrav LH, Heimbach DM, Reus JL, Harnar TJ, Marvin JA (1983) Early excision and grafting vs. nonoperative treatment of burns of indeterminant depth: a randomized prospective study. J Trauma 23(11):1001–1004
5. Godina M, Derganc M, Brcic A (1977) The reliability of clinical assessment of the depth of burns. Burns 4(2):92
6. Haslik W, Kamolz LP, Lumenta DB, Hladik M, Beck H, Frey M (2010) The treatment of deep dermal hand burns: how do we achieve better results? Should we use allogeneic keratinocytes or skin grafts? Burns 36(3):329–334
7. Haslik W, Kamolz LP, Manna F, Hladik M, Rath T, Frey M (2010) Management of full-thickness skin defects in the hand and wrist region: first long-term experiences with the dermal matrix Matriderm. J Plast Reconstr Aesthet Surg 63(2):360–364
8. Haslik W, Kamolz LP, Nathschläger G, Andel H, Meissl G, Frey M (2007) First experiences with the collagen-elastin matrix Matriderm as a dermal substitute in severe burn injuries of the hand. Burns 33(3):364–368
9. Heimbach D, Engrav L, Grube B, Marvin J (1992) Burn depth: a review. World J Surg 16(1):10–15
10. Jackson DM (1953) The diagnosis of the depth of burning. Br J Surg 40:588–596
11. Kamolz LP, Kitzinger HB, Karle B, Frey M (2009) The treatment of hand burns. Burns 35(3):327–337
12. Keck M, Selig HF, Lumenta DB, Kamolz LP, Mittlböck M, Frey M (2012) The use of Suprathel(®) in deep dermal burns: first results of a prospective study. Burns 38(3):388–395
13. Lumenta DB, Kamolz LP, Keck M, Frey M (2011) Comparison of meshed versus MEEK micrografted skin expansion rate: claimed, achieved, and polled results. Plast Reconstr Surg 128(1):40e–41e
14. Lumenta DB, Kamolz LP, Frey M (2009) Adult burn patients with more than 60 % TBSA involved-meek and other techniques to overcome restricted skin harvest availability–the Viennese Concept. J Burn Care Res 30(2):231–242
15. Spurr ED, Shakespeare PG (1990) Incidence of hypertrophic scarring in burned-children. Burns 16(3):179–181
16. Still JM, Law EJ, Belcher K, Thiruvaiyarv D (1996) Decreased length of hospital stay by early excision and grafting of burns. South Med J 89:578–582

Critical Care of Burn Victims Including Inhalation Injury

6

Marc G. Jeschke

6.1 Introduction

There is no greater trauma than major burn injury, which can be classified according to different burn causes and different depths. More than 500,000 burn injuries occur annually in the USA per year [1]. Although most of these burn injuries are minor, approximately 40,000–60,000 burn patients require admission to a hospital or major burn center for appropriate treatment. The devastating consequences of burns have been recognized by the medical community, and significant amounts of resources and research have been dedicated, successfully improving these dismal statistics [2–4]. Specialized burn centers and advances in therapy strategies, based on improved understanding of resuscitation, protocolized and specialized critical care, enhanced wound coverage, more appropriate infection control, improved treatment of inhalation injury, and better support of the hypermetabolic response to injury, have further improved the clinical outcome of this unique patient population over the past years [4, 5]. However, severe burns remain a devastating injury affecting nearly every organ system and leading to significant morbidity and mortality [2–6]. Of all cases, nearly 4,000 people die of complications related to thermal injury [2].

Burn deaths generally occur either immediately after the injury or weeks later as a result of infection/sepsis, multisystem organ failure, or hypermetabolic catabolic responses [5, 7]. Therefore, this chapter is divided into critical care during the early

M.G. Jeschke, MD, PhD, FACS, FCCM, FRCS(C)
Division of Plastic Surgery, Department of Surgery and Immunology,
Ross Tilley Burn Centre, Sunnybrook Health Sciences Centre,
Sunnybrook Research Institute, University of Toronto,
Rm D704, Bayview Ave. 2075, M4N 3M5 Toronto, ON, Canada
e-mail: marc.jeschke@sunnybrook.ca

M.G. Jeschke et al. (eds.), *Burn Care and Treatment*,
DOI 10.1007/978-3-7091-1133-8_6, © Springer-Verlag Wien 2013

phases and later phases. The quality of the complex care of burn patients is directly related to the outcome and survival of burn patients. The key aspects for the care are:

1. *Initial care at the scene and prehospital*: adequate and timely response, evaluation of the burns, treatment of the burn patient, resuscitation, initial pain, and transport
2. *Early hospital phase*: admission to a burn center, escharotomies/fasciotomies, resuscitation, treatment of inhalation injury, and critical care to maintain organ perfusion and function
3. *Later hospital phase*: wound care including burn surgeries, infection control, attenuation of hypermetabolism, and maintaining organ function

In this chapter, we focus on critical care components that have been shown to contribute to increased postburn morbidity and mortality and are typical hallmarks of critical care responses. As Chap. 1 delineated prehospital, fluid, and early management, we will focus on early hospital phase and later hospital phase.

6.2 Initial and Early Hospital Phase

In the initial management, therapeutic goal for these patients is prevention of organ failure, which begins with adequate resuscitation [8–12]. Resuscitation and all current formulas are discussed in detail in Chap. 1. Resuscitation is, however, also one of the key aspects of the early phase in critical care. Once the burn patient is received by the accepting burn center, the patient usually is evaluated and treated in the tub room. This visit includes cleansing, evaluation of burn wounds, possible escharotomies/fasciotomies, intubation including bronchoscopy and diagnosis of inhalation injury, placement of arterial and venous access, Foley catheter, and adequate dressing care. Once these interventions are finished, the central element of critical care is monitoring the vital signs:

- Invasive arterial blood pressure
- Noninvasive blood pressure (not recommended for large burns >40 % TBSA)
- Urine output
- CVP
- Oxygen saturation
- Respiratory rate
- Blood gas with lactate
- Ventilation settings
- Invasive and noninvasive thermodilution catheter (e.g., PiCCO catheter to monitor CO, CI, SVR, SVRI, ETBV, lung water)
- Serum organ marker (liver, kidney, pancreas, endocrine system)
- Central and peripheral tissue perfusion

6.2.1 Blood Pressure

Continuous monitoring of the arterial blood pressure ensures adequate organ perfusion and is a key aspect in the initial postburn phase. In general, a MAP of >60–65 mmHg should be maintained. Chronic hypertensive patients may require a greater MAP which can vary. The most common problem during the first 24–48 h postburn is hypotension with very few patients having hypertension. Adequate MAP and organ perfusion can be achieved by:

- Adequate fluid resuscitation (e.g., Parkland 4 cc/kg/m^2 burn of RL)
- Albumin substitution after 8–12 h postburn if resuscitation fails (5 % albumin 75–125 cc/h)
- Transfusion of PRBC
- Dobutamin if cardiac index is low (5–10 micro/kg/min)
- Vasopressin if patient experiences vasodilation and low MAP (1.2–2.4 IU)
- Norepinephrine or epinephrine persistent and refractory hypotension

If a patient is hypertensive (systolic >200 mmHg or diastolic >120 mmHg) and has signs of over-resuscitation, decrease vasopressors, decrease fluids, and decrease albumin in stages until MAP is targeted. If the patient is on no vasopressors, inotropes, and hypertensive, recommendations are:

- Nitroprusside (>0.5 micro/kg/min)
- Labetalol (10–20 mg)
- Nicardipine (5 mg/h)
- Nifedipine (5 mg sublingual)

6.2.1.1 Resuscitation

Adequate resuscitation is a key element of early burn critical care [8–12]. Maintenance of organ perfusion during burn shock depends upon restoration of intravascular volume. The most common algorithm, the Parkland formula, calculates a total volume of crystalloid to be given over the first 24 h according to 4 cc/kg (patient weight) × %TBSA (total body surface area burnt) [8, 13–15]. In accordance to the American Burn Association (ABA), the resuscitation formula is only to be used as a guideline for resuscitation in burn shock [9–11, 14, 16]. The Parkland formula is deficient in calculating the fluid requirements for resuscitation in patients with large burn size/deeper burns, inhalation injury, delays in resuscitation, alcohol or drug use, as well as those with electrical injury leading to inadequate/inappropriate resuscitation. The endpoints (urine output of 0.5 cc/kg/h, MAP > 65), which traditionally had been used for fluid resuscitation, are not always adequate. With the advent of goal-directed therapy [8, 13–15, 17], it has become apparent that the Parkland formula can underestimate or overestimate fluid requirements. However, with this discovery and efforts to improve fluid resuscitation, patients with severe burns receive far greater crystalloid volumes than predicted by the Parkland formula resulting in "fluid creep" [9, 10, 15, 18] with its inherent complications such as pulmonary edema, pleural effusions, pericardial effusions, abdominal compartment syndrome, extremity compartment syndrome, and conversion of burns to deeper wounds. In addition, increasing fluid requirements in burn patients significantly increased the risk of developing ARDS, pneumonia, bloodstream infections, multiorgan failure, and death [16]. Given the risk of abdominal compartment syndrome with large burn and its dire consequences, intra-abdominal pressure monitoring is therefore recommended in the burns involving more than 30 % TBSA [19].

The initial resuscitation should aim to maintain organ perfusion: urinary output 0.5 ml/h, lack of tachycardia, maintenance of MAP ≥60 mmHg, normal lactate, and base excess levels will generally reflect this global condition [2, 15, 16]. As

Table 6.1 Criteria for assessment of under- and over-resuscitation

Under-resuscitation	Over-resuscitation
Oliguria <0.3 ml/kg/h	Polyuria >1.0 ml/kg/h
Hemoglobin >180 g/l (Ht > 55 %)	Decreasing PaO_2/FiO_2, → pulmonary edema
Natremia >145 mmol/l	Increasing PAPO/PVC
Cardiac index <2 l/min/m²	Rapidly increasing cutaneous edema
SvO_2 <55 %	Fluid delivery > Ivy index (fluid delivery >250 ml/kg BW)
Plasma lactate >2 mmol/l or increasing	Intra-abdominal pressure $P > 20$ mmHg → Intra-abdominal hypertension leading to
Base excess < −5 mmol/l or decreasing	→ Acute renal failure, splanchnic ischemia, transformation of 2–3° burns, compartment syndrome in limbs (↑need for fasciotomies), ↓venous return with hemodynamic failure

mentioned before, the majority of burn surgeons will use the Parkland formula for the first 24 h. It is imperative to look for signs of adequate, over-, and under-resuscitation (Table 6.1).

After 24–48 h, the patients generally become spontaneously hyperdynamic, and the fluid delivery should be drastically reduced, to about 30–40 % of that infused during the first 24 h. The total daily maintenance in terms of fluid requirements can be calculated by

$$\text{Basal fluid } 1{,}500cc\,/\,m^2 + \text{evaporative water loss} \left[(25 + \%\ \text{burn})\text{*}m^2\text{*}24 \right]$$
$$= \text{total maintenance fluid; } m^2 \text{ in meter square}$$

However, calculated fluid balances are difficult to calculate, as they do not take into account the exact amount of exudative losses through the burn wounds (about 0.5–1 l/10 % TBSA/day). The condition may be complicated by the used of fluidized or air beds, which cause an even greater loss of free water. By day 3, the interstitial fluids that have accumulated during the first 24–48 h must be mobilized and excreted. This generally required an active stimulation of diuresis using loop diuretics (generally furosemide) and sometimes in combination with an aldosterone antagonist Aldactone.

6.2.1.2 Albumin

The use of albumin in burn patients is not well defined, and to date no prospective randomized trial in burn patients shows the advantage or disadvantage of albumin administration for burn resuscitation, maintenance, or burn infection/sepsis [10, 20]. A lot of burn care providers believe that albumin has a positive effect in the case of burn resuscitation as a rescue modality. In general, in case of hypoalbuminemia <20 g/l, the colloid osmotic pressure shifts to the extent that fluid is not resorbed, and therefore, fluid stays in the interstitial space enhancing edema formation. We believe that albumin should be used for difficult resuscitations, and we believe that hypoalbuminemia <20 g/l should be corrected to avoid the negative consequences of decreased oncotic pressure.

6.2.1.3 Transfusion

Transfusion guidelines are currently being investigated and most like changed. The gold standard of 100 mg/dl has been questioned, and a large multicenter trial is ongoing and investigates transfusion thresholds 70 vs. 100 mg/dl. Our practice is to target a level of least 70 mg/dl, but if a patient is premorbid with impaired cardiac function or poor oxygen delivery, we consider reaching hemoglobin levels of 80–90 mg/dl.

6.2.1.4 Vasopressors

Vasopressors or inotropes can be used if indicated. Usually during the first 8–12 h, vasopressors should be avoided as vasoconstriction can have adverse effects. However, dobutamine as an inotrope can improve cardiac function if CO or CI is low (<3 l/min/m^2). Classical vasopressors epinephrine and norepinephrine should be used with caution. Vasopressin is becoming a possibility that is currently studied in various trials. In the critical care population, vasopressin did not improve outcome compared to catecholamines. In addition, there are case reports that have no benefit with vasopressin but with an increased incidence of adverse effects, which is usually associated with high doses of vasopressin (>2.4 IU). However, it appears that doses between 1.2 and 2.4 IU are relatively safe and can improve the blood pressure. Our center usually uses vasopressin as a second-line agent. Dopamine, another inotropic agent, is used by some but generally is not widely used for burns.

6.2.2 Urine Output

Urinary output in the acute phase of a burn is indicative of adequate organ perfusion, and the suggested target is 0.5–1 cc/kg/h. In children, UOP is targeted to 1 cc/kg/h. However, UOP is not always adequate and can be affected by the burn itself, infusion of antioxidants during resuscitation, and central or peripheral renal insufficiency.

6.2.3 CVP

CVP is a rough marker for preload and hence filling of the patient. Of importance is that CVP should be measured correctly at the level of the heart with a subclavian or jugular line in place. The range of an adequate CVP in burned adults is 4–8 mmHg, which is 2–6 mmHg in burned children.

6.2.4 Respiration

Respiratory rate, respiratory effort, breath sounds, and skin color reflect oxygenation and provide objective measurements of breathing. A respiratory rate of less than 10 or greater than 60 is a sign of impending respiratory failure. Use of accessory

Table 6.2 Indication for intubation [2, 4]

Criteria	Value
PaO$_2$ (mmHg)	<60
PaCO$_2$ (mmHg)	>50 (acutely)
P/F ratio	<200
Respiratory/ventilatory failure	Impending
Upper airway edema	Severe
Severe facial burn	
Burns over 40 % TBSA	
Clinical signs of severe inhalation injury	

muscles, manifested by supraclavicular, intercostal, subcostal, or sternal retractions, and the presence of grunting or nasal flaring are signs of increased work of breathing. Auscultation of breath sounds provides a clinical determination of tidal volume. Skin color deteriorates from pink to pale, to mottled, and to blue as hypoxemia progresses. These signs must be followed throughout the primary survey to avoid respiratory failure. Patients with probable respiratory failure should receive rapid, aggressive, and definitive airway management (Tables 6.2 and 6.3).

Oral intubation with the largest appropriate endotracheal tube is the preferred method for obtaining airway access and should be accomplished early if impending respiratory failure or ventilatory obstruction is anticipated.

Oxygen saturation in the initial phase but also during the later phase of hospitalization should be over 85–90. Respiratory should be 8–20 in adults and 14–38 in children.

Effective gas exchange should be determined in an arterial blood gas analysis. Targets for good oxygenation as well as organ perfusion are those with pH>7.25.

6.2.4.1 Ventilation Settings

The different modes of ventilation including high-frequency oscillation are all being investigated and tested. Detailed descriptions of the different modes are beyond the scope of this handbook. In short, PEEP is useful in supporting oxygenation. The level of PEEP required should be established by empirical trials and reevaluated on a regular basis. PEEP levels should start at 5 cmH$_2$O and be increased in 2–3 cm increments. PEEP trials should be done to optimize oxygenation and cardiac output. The effectiveness of continuous positive airway pressure (CPAP) or PEEP is related to surface tension abnormalities and the marked tendency for atelectasis in these patients. Pressure control ventilation with permissive hypercapnia is the current preferred method of treatment for ventilated patients. If pulmonary edema continues, the amount of PEEP and of oxygen should be elevated so as to maintain adequate gas exchange. The use of high-frequency oscillating ventilators in the pressure control mode may also result in better removal of airway debris. Low tidal volumes (5–8 ml/kg) with PEEP may be needed to improve oxygenation. Peak flow rates should be adjusted as needed to satisfy patient inspiratory demands. For inspiratory/expiratory (I:E) ratio, the inspiratory time should be long enough to deliver the tidal volume at

Table 6.3 Extubation criteria

In general, early as possible	
Criteria	Value
PaO$_2$/FiO$_2$ (P/F) ratio	>250
Maximum inspiratory pressure (MIP) (cmH$_2$O)	>60
Spontaneous tidal volume (ml/kg)	>5–7
Spontaneous vital capacity (ml/kg)	>15–20
Maximum voluntary ventilation	>Twice the minute volume
Audible leak around the ET tube with cuff deflated	

flow rates that will not result in airway turbulence and high peak airway pressures. The normal I:E ratio is 1:2. This may be adjusted to increase the ratio if oxygenation becomes difficult. Inspired oxygen concentration as a starting point and until the level of hypoxemia is determined; a patient placed on a ventilator should receive an oxygen concentration of 100 %. Decrease the FiO$_2$ as ABGs improve.

Ventilator management (guideline from the American College of Chest physicians) targeted should be an acceptable oxygen saturation; a plateau pressure of greater than 35 cmH$_2$O is cause for concern (clinical conditions that are associated with a decreased chest wall compliance, plateau pressures greater than 35 cmH$_2$O may be acceptable). To accomplish the goal of limiting plateau pressures, PCO$_2$'s should be permitted to rise (permissive hypercapnia) unless other contraindications exist that demand a more normal PCO$_2$ or pH.

6.2.5 Inhalation Injury

Twenty to 30 % of all major burns are associated with a concomitant inhalation injury, with a mortality of 25–50 % when patients required ventilatory support for more than 1 week post-injury [2, 4, 21]. A significant portion of fire-related deaths result not from burn injury but from inhalation of the toxic products of combustion [14, 21–23]. Many of these compounds may act together, so as to increase mortality. This is especially true of carbon monoxide (CO) and hydrogen cyanide (HCN) where a synergism has been found to increase tissue hypoxia and acidosis and may also decrease cerebral oxygen consumption and metabolism. Cyanide (CN) toxicity associated with inhalation injury remains a diagnostic dilemma as markers for CN toxicity (elevated blood lactate, elevated base deficit, or metabolic acidosis) can also represent under-resuscitation, associated trauma, CO poisoning, or hypoxia. Regardless, aggressive resuscitation and administration of 100 % oxygen remains a mainstay of treatment. Controversy remains as to the need for specific antidotes in cyanide poisoning [24]. The use of hydroxocobalamin (a standard of prehospital care in some Europe centers) has not been as widely accepted in North America. There is minimal evidence for the role of CN antidotes in smoke inhalation injury; therefore, aggressive supportive therapy aimed at allowing for the hepatic clearance of cyanide without specific antidotes should be the first line of treatment. Other possible contributing toxic substances are hydrogen chloride (produced by polyvinyl chloride degradation), nitrogen oxide, or aldehydes which can result in pulmonary edema, chemical pneumonitis, or respiratory irritability. Direct thermal damage to the lung is seldom seen except as a result of high-pressure steam, which has 4.000 times the heat-carrying capacity of dry air. Laryngeal reflexes and the efficiency of heat dissipation in the upper airway prevent heat damage to the lung parenchyma.

The clinical course of patients with inhalation injury is divided into three stages:

- First stage: Acute pulmonary insufficiency. Patients with severe lung injuries show acute pulmonary insufficiency from 0 to 36 h after injury with asphyxia, carbon monoxide poisoning, bronchospasm, upper airway obstruction, and parenchymal damage.
- Second stage: Pulmonary edema. This second stage occurs in 5–30 % of patients, usually from 6 to 72 h postburn and is associated with a high mortality rate.
- Third stage: Bronchopneumonia. It appears in 15–60 % of these patients and has a reported mortality of 50–86 %. Bronchopneumonia occurs typically 3–10 days after burn injury and is often associated with the expectoration of large mucus casts formed in the tracheobronchial tree. Those pneumonias appearing in the first few days are usually due to penicillin-resistant Staphylococcus species, whereas after 3–4 days, the changing flora of the burn wound is reflected in the appearance in the lung of gram-negative species, especially Pseudomonas species.

Early detection of bronchopulmonary injury is critical in improving survival after a suspected inhalation injury. The following are the clinical signs [14, 21, 25]:

- History of exposure to smoke in closed space (patients who are stuporous or unconscious).
- Physical findings of facial burns/singed nasal vibrissae/bronchorrhea/sooty sputum/auscultatory findings (wheezing or rales).
- Laboratory findings: hypoxemia and/or elevated levels of carbon monoxide.
- Chest X-ray (insensitive method because admission studies are very seldom abnormal and may remain normal as long as 7 days postburn).
- Bronchoscopy should be the standard diagnostic method on every burn patient. Inhalation injury can be graded using the scale of Gamelli [23]:
  - No inhalation injury or grade 0
  - Absence of carbonaceous deposits, erythema, edema, bronchorrhea, or obstruction
  - *Mild injury or grade I injury*:
    Minor or patchy areas of erythema, carbonaceous deposits in proximal, or distal bronchi any or combination
  - *Moderate injury or grade II injury*:
    Moderate degree of erythema, carbonaceous deposits, and bronchorrhea with or without compromise of the bronchi any or combination
  - *Severe injury or grade III injury*:
    Severe inflammation with friability, copious carbonaceous deposits, bronchorrhea, bronchial obstruction any or combination

– *Massive injury or grade IV injury*:
Evidence of mucosal sloughing, necrosis, endoluminal obliteration any or combination:

- To define parenchymal injury, the most specific method is the 133 Xe lung scanning, which involves intravenous injection of radioactive xenon gas followed by serial chest scintiphotograms. This technique identifies areas of air trapping from small airway partial or total obstruction by demonstrating areas of decreased alveolar gas washout.
- Additionally, pulmonary function test can be performed and could show an increased resistance and decreased flow in those with abnormal 133 Xe scans.

The treatment of the inhalation injury should start immediately (Table 6.4), with the administration of 100 % oxygen via face mask or nasal cannula. This helps reverse the effects of CO poisoning and aids in its clearance, as 100 % oxygen lowers its half-life time from 250 to less than 50 min. Maintenance of the airway is critical. If early evidence of upper airway edema is present, early intubation is required, because the upper airway edema normally increases over 8–12 h. Prophylactic intubation without good indication, however, should not be performed; for intubation criteria, see Tables 6.2 and 6.3.

Several clinical studies have shown that pulmonary edema could not be prevented by fluid restriction. Indeed, fluid resuscitation appropriate for the patients' other needs results in a decrease in lung water, has no adverse effect on pulmonary histology, and improves survival. Although overhydration could increase pulmonary edema, inadequate hydration increases the severity of pulmonary injury by sequestration of polymorphonuclear cells and leads to increased mortality.

Prophylactic antibiotics for inhalation injury are not indicated, but clearly are indicated for documented lung infections. Empiric choices for treatment of pneumonias prior to culture results should include coverage of methicillin-resistant Staphylococcus aureus in the first few days postburn (these develop within the first week after burn) and of gram-negative organisms (especially Pseudomonas or Klebsiella) which mostly occur after 1 week postburn. Systemic antibiotic regimes are based on serially monitored sputum cultures, bronchial washings, or transtracheal aspirates.

The theoretical benefits of corticosteroid therapy include a reduction in mucosal edema, reduced bronchospasm, and the maintenance of surfactant function. However, in several animal and clinical studies, mortality increased with the administration of corticosteroids, and bronchopneumonia showed a more extensive abscess formation. Thus, the use of corticosteroids is contraindicated.

Table 6.4 Pharmacological management

Bronchodilators (albuterol)	Q 2 h
Nebulized heparin	5.000–10.000 units with 3 cc normal saline Q 4 h which alternates with
Nebulized acetylcysteine	20 %, 3 cc Q 4 h
Hypertonic saline induce	Effective coughing
Racemic epinephrine	Reduce mucosal edema

Prognosis: Inhalation injury is one of the most important predictors of morbidity and mortality in burn patients. When present, Inh-Inj increases mortality in up to 15 times [14, 21, 24, 26]. Inh-Inj requires endotracheal intubation, which in turn increases the incidence of pneumonia. As mentioned before, pneumonia is a common complication of Inh-Inj and increases mortality in up to 60 % in these patients. Patients usually recover full pulmonary function, and late complications are not the rule. Complications can be secondary to the Inh-Inj or to the endotracheal or tracheostomy tube. Hyperreactive airways and altered patterns on pulmonary function (obstructive and restrictive) have been described following Inh-Inj. Scarring of the airway can cause stenosis and changes in the voice, requiring voice therapy and occasionally surgery.

6.2.6 Invasive and Noninvasive Thermodilution Catheter (PiCCO Catheter)

A novel approach for burn patients has been the use of thermodilution catheters to determine cardiac function, resistance, and lung water [11, 27, 28]. The use of these catheters may enable focused and algorithm-driven therapy that may improve the resuscitation phase, but as of now there are only few small studies published that do not allow major conclusions. But these systems show promising results to optimize resuscitation [11].

Volume status and cardiac performance are especially difficult to evaluate in the burned victim. In particular, burned extremities may impede the ability to obtain a blood pressure reading by a sphygmomanometer (blood pressure cuff). In these situations, arterial lines, particularly femoral lines, are useful to monitor continuous blood pressure readings. Invasive hemodynamic monitoring via pulmonary artery catheter (PAC) permits the direct and continuous measurement of central venous pressure (CVP), pulmonary capillary wedge pressure, cardiac output (CO), systemic vascular resistance (SVR), oxygen delivery (DO_2), and oxygen consumption (VO_2). PAC-guided therapy has been studied most extensively in trauma and critically ill surgical patients. It has been shown that hemodynamic data derived from the PAC appeared to be beneficial to ascertain cardiovascular performance in certain situations (inadequate noninvasive monitoring, difficulty to define endpoints of resuscitation). However, the general practicability, risk-benefit ratio, and lack of mortality reduction when using PAC have been widely criticized. At the moment, there are no studies in burn patients to provide evidence-based recommendations. In order to overcome the disadvantages of the PAC, less-invasive techniques have been developed.

With transpulmonary thermodilution (TPTD), a cold saline bolus is injected into the central venous circulation, and the subsequent change in blood temperature is picked up by a thermistor-tipped arterial catheter. This is connected to a commercially available device (PiCCO®) that calculates flows and volumes from the dilution curves. In addition to CO and SVR measurement, TPTD allows an estimation of global end-diastolic volume (GEDV) and intrathoracic blood volume (ITBV), both indicators of cardiac preload, and extravascular lung water (EVLW), which is

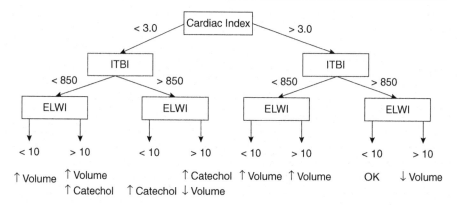

Fig. 6.1 Treatment algorithm to maintain adequate organ perfusion using inotropes, fluid, CI and diuretics (From [11])

a marker of pulmonary edema. The use of TPTD goal-directed therapy based on ITBV and EVLW measurements in critically ill patients has been studied in various prospective trials and showed promising results, none of these is, however, specific for burn patients.

In our center, we use an algorithm to optimize fluid resuscitation and cardiac performance in the acute setting as well as during the ICU stay [11] (Fig. 6.1):

6.2.7 Serum Organ Markers

In our opinion, it is imperative to follow organ function from the initial phase after injury throughout ICU and hospital stay. The most feasible approach is to measure serum markers of organ function or dysfunction/damage. We recommend [4]:
- Cardiac markers: troponin, A- and B-natriuretic peptide, CK
- Liver: AST, ALT, Bili, ALKP
- Pancreas: amylase, lipase
- Kidney: BUN, creatinine
- Hematology: CBC including coagulation, differential including bands
- Hormonal: cortisol including ACTH challenge, thyroid axis, GnRH

For longitudinal observation, it is recommended to obtain admission values and measures values once or twice per week.

6.3 Later Hospital Phase

The later phase includes critical practices to maintain organ function, control infection and sepsis, and alleviate hypermetabolism. This section will focus on maintaining organ function and complication of long-term ICU sequelae as infection and sepsis are discussed in detail in Chap. 5, and hypermetabolism is covered in Chap. 8.

6.3.1 Central Nervous System

Anoxic brain injury used to be the leading cause of death in burn patients, which has been replaced by sepsis and MOF [7]. Adequate resuscitation and early intubation improved mortality in burn patient [12, 14]. However, neurological disturbances are commonly observed in burned patients. The possibility of cerebral edema and raised intracranial pressure must be considered during the early fluid resuscitation phase, especially in the case of associated brain injury or high-voltage electrical injury. Inhalation of neurotoxic chemicals, of carbon monoxide, or of hypoxic encephalopathy may adversely affect the central nervous system as well as arterial hypertension [14, 21, 22, 24]. Other factors include hypo-/hypernatremia, hypovolemic shock, sepsis, antibiotic overdosage (e.g., penicillin), and possible oversedation or withdrawal effects of sedative drugs. If increased intracranial pressure is suspected, neurosurgery needs to consulted and most likely bolt are place and therapy initiated to decreased intracranial pressure.

In general, severe burn injury is associated with nonspecific atrophy of the brain that normally resolves over time. No intervention is needed.

Pain and anxiety will generally require rather large doses of opioids and sedatives (benzodiazepines mainly). Continuous infusion regimens will generally be successful in maintaining pain within acceptable ranges. Sedatives and analgesics should be targeted to appropriate sedation and pain scales (SAS or VAS scores four appear optimal), thus preventing the sequelae associated with oversedation and opioid creep, namely, fluid creep and effects on the central and peripheral cardiovascular system [18]. Therefore, consideration should be given to the use of NMDA receptor antagonist, such as ketamine or gabapentin, who have important opioid-sparing effects to decrease the need for opioids and benzodiazepines [2, 4]. We find multimodal pain management combining a long-acting opioid for background pain, a short-acting opioid for procedures, an anxiolytic, an NSAID, acetaminophen, and gabapentin for neuropathic pain control [2, 4] used at our institution targeted to SAS (sedation score) and VAS (visual analog scale) scores provides adequate analgesia and sedation.

6.3.1.1 Intensive Care Unit-Acquired Weakness

Survival and organ function have been the main outcome measures for burn patients; however, recently long-term outcomes move into the focus of burn care providers. A significant component of long-term outcomes include the peripheral nervous system and muscular system which manifest as neuromyopathy. The importance of positioning and prevention of peripheral nerve compression is well known and ingrained in the daily practices of most critical care units. The main risk factors for neuropathy include multiple organ failure, muscular inactivity, hyperglycemia, use of corticosteroids, and neuromuscular blockers. In a recent publication by de Jonghe and Bos [29], early identification and treatment of conditions leading to multiple organ failure, especially sepsis and septic shock, avoiding unnecessary deep sedation and excessive hyperglycemia, promoting early mobilization, and weighing the risk and benefits of corticosteroids might reduce the incidence and severity of ICU-acquired weakness.

6.3.1.2 Thermal Regulation

Temperature regulation is altered with a "resetting" of the hypothalamic temperature above normal values [30–32]. The teleological advantage of maintaining an elevated core temperature following burn injury is not fully understood, but major burns destroy the insulating properties of the skin, while the patients strive for a temperature of 38.0–38.5 °C. Sometimes it is difficult to differentiate elevated temperatures due to a central reset or due to other causes such as infection or fever. Our protocol calls for cultures if temperatures are persistently over 39 °C.

Catecholamine production contributes to the changes in association with several cytokines, including interleukin-1 and interleukin-6. Any attempt to lower the basal temperature by external means will result in augmented heat loss, thus increasing metabolic rate. Ambient temperature should be maintained between 28 and 33 °C to limit heat loss and the subsequent hypermetabolic response [3]. Metabolic rate is increased as a consequence of several factors such as the catecholamine burst, the thermal effects of proinflammatory cytokines, and evaporative losses from the wounds, which consume energy, causing further heat loss. The evaporation causes extensive fluid losses from the wounds, approximating 4,000 ml/m^2/%TBSA burns [2, 4]. Every liter of evaporated fluid corresponds to a caloric expenditure of about 600 kcal.

Beside hyperthermia another very important contributor to poor outcome is hypothermia. Burn patients frequently experience hypothermia (defined as core temperature below 35 °C) on admission, on the ICU, during OR, and during sepsis [2, 4]. Time to recover from hypothermia has been shown to be predictive of outcome in adults, with time to revert to normothermia being longer in non-survivors. Considering that hypothermia favors infections and delays wound healing, the maintenance of perioperative normothermia is of utmost importance. Tools include warming the ambient room temperature, intravenous fluid warming systems, and warming blankets. The temperature of the bed should be set at 38 ± 0.5 °C. However, this is contraindicated in the febrile patient, as it complicates fluid therapy due to largely unpredictable free water losses and respiratory management due to the supine position. The patient may require additional 1–4 l of free water per day (as D5W IV or enteral free water) to prevent dehydration. These additional requirements are difficult to assess in absence of bed-integrated weight scales. This further exposes the gut to dehydration with subsequent constipation.

6.3.2 Heart

The typical complication in severely burned patients is cardiomyopathy requiring inotrope therapy, which was discussed above.

Another complication that can occur is cardiac ischemia. Ischemic events can lead to a manifest heart or to temporary cardiac ischemia. If a heart attack occurs (ECG, Trops, CK, clinical symptoms), cardiology should be immediately involved and guide therapy that usually includes aspirin, beta-blocker, nitro. Cardiology can also refer the patient to interventional cardiology for an angio.

6.3.3 Lung

Pulmonary complications in the early phase are pulmonary edema and inhalation injury that was discussed above. A pulmonary problem that occurs during ICU or hospital stay is VAP (ventilation-associated pneumonia) and ARDS.

6.3.3.1 Ventilator-Associated Pneumonia

The ABA guidelines for prevention, diagnosis, and treatment of ventilator-associated pneumonia (VAP) in burn patients were published in 2009 [15, 33]. The guidelines are as follows:

- Mechanically ventilated burn patients are at high risk for developing VAP, with the presence of inhalation injury as a unique risk factor in this patient group.
- VAP prevention strategies should be used in mechanically ventilated burn patients.
- Clinical diagnosis of VAP can be challenging in mechanically ventilated burn patients where systemic inflammation and acute lung injury are prevalent. Therefore, a quantitative strategy, when available, is the preferable method to confirm the diagnosis of VAP.
- An 8-day course of targeted antibiotic therapy is generally sufficient to treat VAP; however, resistant Staphylococcus aureus and gram-negative bacilli may require longer treatment duration.
- Any effort should be made to reduce length of intubation.

Our policy is to administer antibiotics according to the length of hospitalization. Patients admitted within the past 5 days should be started on an empiric regimen of

Ceftriaxone 1 g iv q24h +/− cloxacillin 1–2 g iv q4–6 h

Penicillin Allergy:

Levofloxacin 750 mg iv/po q24h

Late Phase (admitted >5 days):

Piperacillin/tazobactam 4.5 g iv q6h (renal dosing required)

+/− vancomycin 1 g iv q12h (with pre- and post-levels around the third dose)

Penicillin Allergy:

Tobramycin 2 mg/kg q8h (in nonobese patients with crcl >70 ml/min) + vancomycin 1 g iv q12h (with pre- and post-levels around the third dose)

Or

Meropenem 500 mg iv q6h (renal dosing required)

6.3.4 Liver/GI

Severe burn injury causes numerous metabolic alterations, including hyperglycemia, lipolysis, and protein catabolism [3, 6, 34]. These changes can induce multiorgan failure and sepsis leading to significant morbidity and mortality [34–36]. Liver plays a significant role in mediating survival and recovery of burn patients, and preexisting liver disease is directly associated with adverse clinical outcomes following burn injury [37–39]. In the study by Price et al. in 2007, they demonstrated that preexisting liver disease increased mortality risk from 6 to 27 %, indicating that liver impairment worsens the prognosis in patients with thermal injury. Severe burn also directly induces hepatic dysfunction and damage, delaying recovery. More recently, work by Jeschke et al. (2009) and Song et al. (2009) has shed light on the mechanism of the hepatic dysfunction following thermal injury, mainly by the upregulation of the ER stress response, and increased cell death contributing to compromised hepatic function postburn [40–45]. Thus, one must not only be cognizant of the significant deleterious effects of hepatic dysfunction in the thermally injured patient as it has significant consequence in terms of multiorgan failure, morbidity, and subsequent mortality of these patients but also focus on therapeutic modalities to alter this response and possibly improve outcome.

6.3.4.1 GI Complications/GI Prophylaxis/Enteral Nutrition

The effect of thermal injury on the gastrointestinal system was identified in 1970 by Dr Basal Pruitt with the description of Curling's ulcer. During the initial hours, splanchnic blood flow is reduced, except for flow to the adrenals and to the liver. Poorly perfused organs shift toward anaerobic metabolism leading to acidosis. Adequate fluid resuscitation restores perfusion to a great extent. But with overenthusiastic fluid delivery, increasing intra-abdominal pressures and consequently abdominal compartment syndrome (ACS) becomes a matter of concern in both adult and pediatric burn patients [19, 46]. The Ivy index (250 ml/kg fluid resuscitation) is a cutoff value beyond which trouble is nearly certain. Abdominal pressures start rising, soon reaching the "gray zone" of 15–20 mmHg, and then the danger zone >20 mmHg, beyond which medical measures must be taken to reduce the IAP to avoid splanchnic organ ischemia. IAP monitoring is essential for TBSA >30 %. Abdominal compartment syndrome is a complication that is associated with high mortality, and in general, laparotomy should be avoided. Abdominal pressure should be controlled by diuresis, sedation, and even paralytics if needed. If the abdomen is burned checkerboard, escharotomies need to be performed.

The gut is extremely vulnerable to changes in perfusion and nutrition. Even short ischemia can lead to gut atrophy associated with several complications. Early enteral feeding should be initiated no later than 12 h after injury. The benefits of this strategy are numerous: increasing blood flow to the splanchnic compartment before edema makes it impossible, maintaining pyloric function, maintaining intestinal motility, and reducing significantly infectious complications. Current recommendations are to place a nasogastric feeding tube as well as post-pyloric feeding tube.

During the initial phase postburn as well as after each ischemia-reperfusion hit, gastrointestinal function, including pyloric function, is vastly depressed. A true paralytic ileus will ensue for many days if the gastrointestinal tract is not used. Opiates and sedatives further depress the gastrointestinal function, and constipation is frequent and may become critical with the development of ileus and intestinal obstruction by feces. Prevention should be initiated from admission using fiber-containing enteral diets, lactulose (osmotic cathartic), and enemas when the other measures have failed. Regular bowel movements need to be diligently monitored.

Gut complications may be life threatening: in addition to the already mentioned ACS and constipation, the patients may develop Ogilvie syndrome, ischemic and non-ischemic bowel necrosis, and intestinal hemorrhage. A careful tight supervision of bowel function with daily examinations is therefore mandatory, particularly in perioperative periods with intraoperative hemorrhage leading to hypovolemia, which exposes the patient to gut hypoperfusion and their threatened complications.

Stress ulcer prophylaxis is mandatory, usually by H2-blockers (ranitidine) or proton pump inhibitors since the bleeding risk is elevated in burn injuries and may be life threatening.

6.3.4.2 Micronutrients and Antioxidants

Critically ill burned patients are characterized by a strong oxidative stress, an intense inflammatory response, and a hypermetabolic state that can last months. Trace element (TE) deficiencies have repeatedly been described. The complications observed in major burns such as infections and delayed wound healing can be partly attributed to TE deficiencies [47, 48]. Plasma TE concentrations are low as a result of TE losses in biological fluids, low intakes, dilution by fluid resuscitation, and redistribution from plasma to tissues mediated by the inflammatory response. The large exudative losses cause negative TE balances. Intravenous supplementation trials show that early substitution improves recovery (IV doses: Cu 3.5 mg/day, Se 400–500 mcg/day, Zn 40 mg/day), reduces infectious complications (particularly nosocomial pneumonia), normalizes thyroid function, improves wound healing, and shortens hospital length of stay. The mechanisms underlying these improvements are a combination of antioxidant effects (particularly of selenium through restoration of glutathione peroxidase activity) and also immune (Cu, Se, Zn) and anabolic effects (Zn particularly).

High vitamin C requirements after major burns were identified already in the 1940s and have been confirmed since then. Very interesting studies by Tanaka et al. in 2000 and Kremer in 2010 demonstrated that high doses of vitamin C administered during the first 24 h after a major injury reduced the capillary leak, probably through antioxidant mechanisms, resulting in significant reductions in fluid resuscitation requirements [49, 50].

6.3.5 Renal

Acute renal failure (ARF) is a major complication of burn injury. The incidence of ARF in burned patients ranges from 1.2 to 20 % and the incidence of ARF requiring renal replacement therapy (RRT) from 0.7 to 14.6 % [8, 51–53]. Although ARF is relatively rare, early diagnosis is important, as the mortality of burn patients with manifest ARF has been reported around 50 % [51]. Applying the RIFLE classification to burn patients, Coca et al. found that the incidence of acute kidney injury was 27 %, and it carried with it a mortality rate of 73 % in the patients with the most severe acute kidney injury (requiring dialysis).

Burn-related ARF can be divided into early and late ARF, depending on the time of onset with each having different etiologies [53, 54]. Early ARF occurs during the first 5 days postburn, and its main causes are hypovolemia, hypotonia, and myoglobinuria. Prevention focuses on early aggressive fluid resuscitation and escharotomies/fasciotomies. Late ARF begins more than 5 days postburn and is usually multifactorial (generally caused by sepsis and/or nephrotoxic antibiotics) [54]. Regardless of the cause, there is strong evidence that renal replacement therapy (RRT) should be instituted as early as possible in burn patients with renal dysfunction before the traditional criteria for RRT have been established. Further to the discussion of RRT is the choice in mode of delivery. CRRT (continuous renal replacement therapy) offers several potential advantages in the management of severe acute renal failure in burn patients. It is slow and continuous, consequently allowing for very efficient metabolic clearance and ultrafiltration of fluids while minimizing hemodynamic compromise, thus allowing for ongoing optimization of fluid and metabolic management. Hemodialysis is surely a viable option if the patient tolerates it. In children, an alternative is peritoneal dialysis with placement of a Tenckhoff catheter.

6.3.6 Hormonal (Thyroid, Adrenal, Gonadal)

In the postburn state, pronounced hormonal and metabolic changes take place [3, 6], starting immediately after injury. There is a tremendous increase in stress hormones after major burns, the increase being particularly marked during the first 2–3 weeks, but the alterations will persist for months and even years [37]. In response to the afferent stimuli from the burn wound, an intense sympathoadrenal response is elicited. Catecholamine secretion contributes to arterial pressure maintenance and also to a massive increase in cardiac afterload. The concentration of epinephrine and norepinephrine remains elevated for several days after injury and contributes to the integrated neuroendrocrine stress response. Cortisol increases markedly, and the intensity of the response is modulated by optimization of pain control with good analgesia [6, 37]. As with many other hormones, the circadian rhythm also changes. Aldosterone levels increase for several days. ACTH response frequently parallels the cortisol levels and tends to be elevated for a few weeks. The increase in plasma rennin activity and aldosterone persists for several weeks.

A patient suffering from infection/sepsis or persistent hypotension should be considered for possible adrenal insufficiency. The current guidelines call for a baseline cortisol level, and if that level is low, an ACTH challenge test should be performed to rule out insufficiency. If an adrenal insufficiency is present, low dose cortisol should be given.

Glucagon concentration is also increased after burn injury, contributing heavily to the hypermetabolic response, while insulin tends to remain within normal values, being paradoxically normal while plasma glucose concentration is elevated.

The thyroid axis exhibits major abnormalities in the patients with major burns. The most constant finding is a "low T3 syndrome": TSH is generally normal, with low T3 levels and T4 levels in the low-normal values, with elevated rT3 levels reflecting an altered deiodination at the hepatic level. If a low T3 is present, there are two options: to administer selenium because selenium deficiency is associated with low T3 levels, and/or thyroid hormone should be replaced.

Postburn the gonadal axis is depressed in any patient with major burns. In men, postburn changes in testosterone and 17beta-estradiol are greater than in females, even during the first days. Plasma testosterone also decreases steeply in limited burn injury. The alterations last at least 4–5 weeks, but may persist for months in critically ill burned patients. The changes seem proportional to the severity of burns. A decreased pituitary stimulation causes lowered hormonal secretions from the testes. This change contributes to the low anabolic response and opens substitution perspectives. LH is more or less normal, LH-RH is decreased, FSH is low, and prolactin is low to elevated.

In premenopausal females, amenorrhea is a nearly universal phenomenon, despite a near normal 17beta-estradiol plasma concentration. Progesterone levels remain very low for many months after injury. Testosterone response is very different from that of males, with nearly normal concentrations in young females, and normal response to ACTH elicits an increase in testosterone, while it decreases it men. Prolactin levels are also higher than seen in men.

In children, despite adequate nutritional support, severe thermal injury leads to decreased anabolic hormones over a prolonged period of time [37]. These changes contribute to stunting of growth observed after major burns. Female patients have significantly increased levels of anabolic hormones, which are associated with decreased proinflammatory mediators and hypermetabolism, leading to a significantly shorter ICU length of stay compared with male patients

6.3.7 Electrolyte Disorders

Burns is a condition where nearly any electrolyte abnormality can be observed. The causes for these disturbances are many and include fluid resuscitation with crystalloids, exudative and evaporative losses, impaired renal regulation, and responses to counter regulatory hormones.

6.3.7.1 Sodium

During the first 24 h, patients receive major amounts of sodium with their fluid resuscitation. Sodium accumulates in the interstitial space with edema. Despite this, hypernatremia occurring during the first 24 h reflects under-resuscitation and should be treated with additional fluid. Thereafter, mobilization of this fluid during the first weeks frequently results in hypernatremia, and its resolution requires free water. Hypernatremia may also result from persistent evaporative losses from the wounds, particularly in case of treatment on a fluidized bed (contraindicated with severe hypernatremia) or in case of fever. Hypernatremia may also herald a septic episode.

6.3.7.2 Chloride

During the early resuscitation and the surgical debridements of the burn wound, the patients tend to receive significant amounts of NaCl resulting in hyperchloremic acidosis. The excess chloride is difficult to handle for the kidney, but the condition is generally resolved without further intervention.

6.3.7.3 Phosphate and Magnesium

Burns have high requirements for phosphate and magnesium in absence of renal failure. Those requirements start early and are largely explained by two mechanisms: large exudative losses and increased urinary excretion associated with acute protein catabolism and stress response. Stimulation of sodium excretion is usually required and can usually be achieved by the simultaneous administration of free water (D5W IV or enteral water) along with furosemide with or without thiazide diuretics.

6.3.7.4 Calcium

Total plasma calcium concentration consists of three fractions: 15 % is bound to multiple anions (sulfate, phosphate, lactate, citrate), about 40 % is bound to albumin in a ratio of 0.2 mmol/l of calcium per 10 g/l of albumin, and the remaining 45 % circulating as physiologically active ionized calcium. Calcium metabolism is tightly regulated. As albumin levels vary widely in burns and only ionized calcium is biologically active, only ionized calcium is a true indicator of status, as total plasma calcium determination is not a reliable indicator of calcium status: the use of conversion formula is unreliable:

$$[Ca] \text{ calculated} = \text{total } [Ca] \text{ measured} + (0.2 \times (45 - [albumin]))$$

Hypocalcemia may occur during the early resuscitation phase or in the context of massive perioperative blood transfusion and requires intravenous supplementation using any form of available intravenous calcium formulation. Hypercalcemia remains a poorly recognized cause of acute renal failure in patients with major burns that occurs as early as 3 weeks after injury. The triad of hypercalcemia, arterial hypertension, and acute renal failure is well known in other critical illnesses, while the association of hypercalcemia and renal failure in patients with major burns is much less reported in the literature. In a recent retrospective study, hypercalcemia was shown to occur in 19 % of the burned patients with hospital lengths of stay of more than 28 days and was noted to be associated with an increased mortality. Hypercalcemia may also occur in patients with smaller burns requiring a stay of more than 20 days in the ICU. Ionized calcium determination enabled earlier detection, while using total calcium determination "with albumin correction" was only slightly sensitive, as shown by normal corrected values in 15 cases with ionized hypercalcemia. Treatment of hypercalcemia includes hydration, volume expansion, and early mobilization. As most causes of severe hypercalcemia depend on increased osteoclast activation, drugs that decrease bone turnover are effective. The treatment of choice in cases that do not resolve with the simple measures relies on the bisphosphonates, pamidronate disodium, and zoledronic acid, which are available in intravenous forms. In burned children, acute intravenous pamidronate administration has been shown to help preserve bone mass, achieving a sustained therapeutic effect on bone [55]. An alternative treatment of the latter in burns includes anabolic agents such as oxandrolone [56]. The bisphosphonates have been advocated in the prevention of heterotrophic ossification, a complication that occurs in 1.2 % of burn patients.

6.3.8 Bone Demineralization and Osteoporosis

Due to the substantial alterations of calcium and phosphorus metabolism, bone formation is reduced both in adults and children when burns exceed 40 % TBSA. Bone mineral density is significantly lower in burned children compared with the same age normal children. Girls have improved bone mineral content and percent fat compared with boys [6, 57, 58]. The consequences are increased risk of fractures, decreased growth velocity, and stunting. The bone is affected by various means: alteration of mineral metabolism, elevated cytokine and corticosteroid levels, decreased growth hormone (GH), nutritional deficiencies, and intraoperative immobilization. Cytokines contribute to the alterations, particularly interleukin-1beta and interleukin-6, both of which are greatly increased in burns and stimulate osteoblast-mediated bone resorption. The increased cortisol production in thermal injury leads to decreased bone formation, and the low GH levels fail to promote bone formation [59], further exacerbating the situation. Various studies suggest that immobilization plays a significant role in the pathogenesis of burn-associated bone disease. Alterations of magnesium and calcium homeostasis constitute another cause. Hypocalcemia and hypomagnesemia are constant findings, and ionized calcium levels remain low for weeks. The alterations are partly explained by large exudative magnesium and phosphorus losses. A close monitoring of ionized calcium, magnesium, and inorganic phosphate levels is mandatory, since burn patients usually require substantial supplementation by intravenous or enteral routes.

6.3.9 Coagulation and Thrombosis Prophylaxis

The coagulation and hematologic system is profoundly affected by a burn, and the associated changes vary from depletion to overproduction. These acute phase responses are normal for a burn injury and usually require no major or only minor intervention. Hematological alterations observed after burns are complex and can last for several months and can be summarized as follows:
- During the early phase after burns, fibrin split products increase.
- Dilution and consumption explain the early low PT values.
- The coagulation cascade is activated.
- Fibrin, factors V, and VIII increase as part of acute phase response.
- Antithrombin deficiency is frequent.
- Thrombocytosis develops when wounds are closing.

The risk of deep venous thrombosis and of pulmonary embolism is at least as high as in any other surgical condition. In our experience, 13 % of patients develop some form of thrombotic complication. Specific risk factors include central venous lines, prolonged bed rest, and an intense inflammatory state. Prophylaxis should be started from admission. Interruptions for surgery should be reduced to minimum and discussed with the surgical team.

Conclusion

The management of the critically ill thermally injured patient can be very complex. The treatment modalities can remain at times controversial, as there is a lack of high-level evidence. There have been many advances in the field of the critical care of the thermally injured patient, which would benefit from large-scale multicenter trials. This brief chapter highlights few of the important nuances in the care of these patients and places emphasis on the need for intricate support for the all organ systems in order to improve morbidity and mortality.

References

1. WHO (2002) A graphical overview of the global burden of injuries. The injury chart book, vol 29. WHO, Geneva
2. Herndon DN (2007) Treatment of infection in burns. In: Herndon DN (ed) Total burn care, 3rd edn. Saunders Elsevier, Philadelphia
3. Herndon DN, Tompkins RG (2004) Support of the metabolic response to burn injury. Lancet 363(9424):1895–1902
4. Jeschke MG et al (2012) Handbook of burns, vol 1. Springer, Wien New York
5. Kraft R et al (2012) Burn size and survival probability in paediatric patients in modern burn care: a prospective observational cohort study. Lancet 379(9820):1013–1021
6. Jeschke MG et al (2008) Pathophysiologic response to severe burn injury. Ann Surg 248(3):387–401
7. Williams FN et al (2009) The leading causes of death after burn injury in a single pediatric burn center. Crit Care 13(6):R183
8. Barrow RE, Jeschke MG, Herndon DN (2000) Early fluid resuscitation improves outcomes in severely burned children. Resuscitation 45(2):91–96
9. Greenhalgh DG (2007) Burn resuscitation. J Burn Care Res 28(4):555–565
10. Greenhalgh DG (2010) Burn resuscitation: the results of the ISBI/ABA survey. Burns 36(2):176–182
11. Kraft R et al. (2012) Optimized fluid management improves outcomes of pediatric burn patients. J Surg Res 2012 June 6 Epub first
12. Wolf SE et al (1997) Mortality determinants in massive pediatric burns. An analysis of 103 children with >or=80 % TBSA burns (> or =70 % full-thickness). Ann Surg 225(5):554–565; discussion 565–569
13. Greenhalgh DG et al (2007) American Burn Association consensus conference to define sepsis and infection in burns. J Burn Care Res 28(6):776–790
14. Latenser BA (2009) Critical care of the burn patient: the first 48 hours. Crit Care Med 37(10):2819–2826
15. Pham TN, Cancio LC, Gibran NS (2008) American Burn Association practice guidelines burn shock resuscitation. J Burn Care Res 29(1):257–266

16. Klein MB et al (2007) The association between fluid administration and outcome following major burn: a multicenter study. Ann Surg 245(4):622–628
17. Rivers E et al (2001) Early goal-directed therapy in the treatment of severe sepsis and septic shock. N Engl J Med 345:1368–1377
18. Saffle JI (2007) The phenomenon of "fluid creep" in acute burn resuscitation. J Burn Care Res 28(3):382–395
19. Ivy ME et al (2000) Intra-abdominal hypertension and abdominal compartment syndrome in burn patients. J Trauma 49(3):387–391
20. Faraklas I et al (2011) Colloid normalizes resuscitation ratio in pediatric burns. J Burn Care Res 32(1):91–97
21. Palmieri TL et al (2009) Inhalation injury in children: a 10 year experience at Shriners Hospitals for Children. J Burn Care Res 30(1):206–208
22. Sheridan RL, Hess D (2009) Inhaled nitric oxide in inhalation injury. J Burn Care Res 30(1):162–164
23. Endorf FW, Gamelli RL (2007) Inhalation injury, pulmonary perturbations, and fluid resuscitation. J Burn Care Res 28(1):80–83
24. Erdman AR (2007) Is hydroxocobalamin safe and effective for smoke inhalation? Searching for guidance in the haze. Ann Emerg Med 49(6):814–816
25. Finnerty CC, Herndon DN, Jeschke MG (2007) Inhalation injury in severely burned children does not augment the systemic inflammatory response. Crit Care 11(1):R22
26. Barrow RE et al (2005) Mortality related to gender, age, sepsis, and ethnicity in severely burned children. Shock 23(6):485–487
27. Branski LK et al (2011) Transpulmonary thermodilution for hemodynamic measurements in severely burned children. Crit Care 15(2):R118
28. Kuntscher MV et al (2002) Transcardiopulmonary vs pulmonary arterial thermodilution methods for hemodynamic monitoring of burned patients. J Burn Care Rehabil 23(1):21–26
29. de Jonge E, Bos MM (2009) Patients with cancer on the ICU: the times they are changing. Crit Care 13(2):122
30. Gore DC et al (2003) Influence of fever on the hypermetabolic response in burn-injured children. Arch Surg 138(2):169–174; discussion 174
31. Hogan BK et al (2012) Correlation of American Burn Association sepsis criteria with the presence of bacteremia in burned patients admitted to the intensive care unit. J Burn Care Res 33(3):371–378
32. Murray CK et al (2007) Evaluation of white blood cell count, neutrophil percentage, and elevated temperature as predictors of bloodstream infection in burn patients. Arch Surg 142(7):639–642
33. Mosier MJ et al (2011) Early enteral nutrition in burns: compliance with guidelines and associated outcomes in a multicenter study. J Burn Care Res 32(1):104–109
34. Williams FN et al (2009) Modulation of the hypermetabolic response to trauma: temperature, nutrition, and drugs. J Am Coll Surg 208(4):489–502
35. Pereira C, Murphy K, Herndon D (2004) Outcome measures in burn care. Is mortality dead? Burns 30(8):761–771
36. Pereira CT et al (2006) Age-dependent differences in survival after severe burns: a unicentric review of 1,674 patients and 179 autopsies over 15 years. J Am Coll Surg 202(3):536–548
37. Jeschke MG et al (2011) Long-term persistance of the pathophysiologic response to severe burn injury. PLoS One 6(7):e21245
38. Jeschke MG (2009) The hepatic response to thermal injury: is the liver important for postburn outcomes? Mol Med 15(9–10):337–351
39. Price LA et al (2007) Liver disease in burn injury: evidence from a national sample of 31,338 adult patients. J Burns Wounds 7:e1
40. Jeschke MG et al (2011) Insulin protects against hepatic damage postburn. Mol Med 17(5–6):516–522
41. Gauglitz GG et al (2010) Post-burn hepatic insulin resistance is associated with endoplasmic reticulum (ER) stress. Shock 33(3):299–305

42. Song J et al (2009) Severe burn-induced endoplasmic reticulum stress and hepatic damage in mice. Mol Med 15(9–10):316–320
43. Jeschke MG et al (2009) Calcium and Er stress mediate hepatic apoptosis after burn injury. J Cell Mol Med 13:1857–1865
44. Jeschke MG, Mlcak RP, Herndon DN (2007) Morphologic changes of the liver after a severe thermal injury. Shock 28(2):172–177
45. Jeschke MG et al (2007) Changes in liver function and size after a severe thermal injury. Shock 28(2):172–177
46. Ivy ME et al (1999) Abdominal compartment syndrome in patients with burns. J Burn Care Rehabil 20(5):351–353
47. Baxter CR (1987) Metabolism and nutrition in burned patients. Compr Ther 13(1):36–42
48. Medlin S (2012) Nutrition for wound healing. Br J Nurs 21(12):S11–S12, S14–15
49. Kremer T et al (2010) High-dose vitamin C treatment reduces capillary leakage after burn plasma transfer in rats. J Burn Care Res 31(3):470–479
50. Tanaka H et al (2000) Reduction of resuscitation fluid volumes in severely burned patients using ascorbic acid administration: a randomized, prospective study. Arch Surg 135(3):326–331
51. Chrysopoulo MT et al (1999) Acute renal dysfunction in severely burned adults. J Trauma 46(1):141–144
52. Jeschke MG et al (1998) Mortality in burned children with acute renal failure. Arch Surg 133(7):752–756
53. Kallinen O et al (2012) Multiple organ failure as a cause of death in patients with severe burns. J Burn Care Res 33(2):206–211
54. Holm C et al (1999) Acute renal failure in severely burned patients. Burns 25(2):171–178
55. Przkora R et al (2006) Body composition changes with time in pediatric burn patients. J Trauma 60(5):968–971; discussion 971
56. Przkora R, Herndon DN, Suman OE (2007) The effects of oxandrolone and exercise on muscle mass and function in children with severe burns. Pediatrics 119(1):e109–e116
57. Jeschke MG et al (2005) Endogenous anabolic hormones and hypermetabolism: effect of trauma and gender differences. Ann Surg 241(5):759–767; discussion 767–768
58. Jeschke MG et al (2008) Gender differences in pediatric burn patients: does it make a difference? Ann Surg 248(1):126–136
59. Przkora R et al (2006) Beneficial effects of extended growth hormone treatment after hospital discharge in pediatric burn patients. Ann Surg 243(6):796–801; discussion 801–803

Nutrition of the Burned Patient and Treatment of the Hypermetabolic Response

7

Marc G. Jeschke

7.1   Introduction

Advances in therapy strategies, based on improved understanding of resuscitation, enhanced wound coverage, more appropriate infection control, and improved treatment of inhalation injury, improved the clinical outcome of burn patients over the past years [1, 2]. However, severe burns remain a devastating injury affecting nearly every organ system and leading to significant morbidity and mortality [2]. One of the main contributors to adverse outcome of this patient population is the profound stress-induced hypermetabolic response, associated with severe alteration in glucose, lipid, and amino acid metabolism [1, 3–5] (Fig. 7.1).

M.G. Jeschke, MD, PhD, FACS, FCCM, FRCS(C)
Division of Plastic Surgery, Department of Surgery and Immunology,
Ross Tilley Burn Centre, Sunnybrook Health Sciences Centre,
Sunnybrook Research Institute, University of Toronto,
Rm D704, Bayview Ave. 2075, M4N 3M5, Toronto, ON, Canada
e-mail: marc.jeschke@sunnybrook.ca

M.G. Jeschke et al. (eds.), *Burn Care and Treatment*,
DOI 10.1007/978-3-7091-1133-8_7, © Springer-Verlag Wien 2013

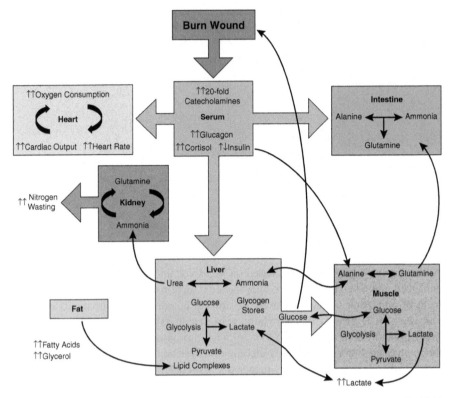

Fig. 7.1 Complexity of the post-burn hypermetabolic response. From Williams FN JACS 2009 April 208(4):489–502

7.2 Post-Burn Hypermetabolism

A hallmark for severely burned patients is the hypermetabolic response that is not only very profound but also extremely complex and most likely induced by stress and inflammation [1, 3–5]. The cause of this response is not entirely defined, but it has been suggested that sustained increases in catecholamine, glucocorticoid, glucagon, and dopamine secretion are involved in initiating the cascade of events leading to the acute hypermetabolic response with its ensuing catabolic state [6–15]. In addition, cytokines, endotoxin, neutrophil-adherence complexes, reactive oxygen species, nitric oxide, and coagulation as well as complement cascades have also been implicated in regulating this response to burn injury [16]. Once these cascades are initiated, their mediators and by-products appear to stimulate the persistent and increased metabolic rate associated with altered glucose, lipid, and amino acid metabolism seen after severe burn injury [17] (Fig. 7.1).

The metabolic changes post-burn occur in two distinct patterns of metabolic regulation following injury [18]:

1. *The first phase occurs within the first 48 h of injury and has classically been called the "ebb phase"* [18, 19], characterized by decreases in cardiac output,

oxygen consumption, and metabolic rate as well as impaired glucose tolerance associated with its hyperglycemic state.

2. The metabolic response then gradually increases within the first 5 days post-injury to a plateau phase and then to flow phase, which is characteristically associated with hyperdynamic circulation and the above-mentioned hypermetabolic state. Insulin release during this time period was found to be twice that of controls in response to glucose load [20, 21], and plasma glucose levels are markedly elevated, indicating the development of an insulin resistance [22, 23]. In addition, lipolysis is tremendously increased leading to increased free fatty acids and triglycerides. Current understanding has been that these metabolic alterations resolve soon after complete wound closure. However, recent studies found that the hypermetabolic response to burn injury lasts significantly longer; we found in recent studies that sustained hypermetabolic alterations post-burn, indicated by persistent elevations of total urine cortisol levels, serum cytokines, catecholamines, and basal energy requirements, were accompanied by impaired glucose metabolism and insulin sensitivity that persisted for up to 3 years after the initial burn injury [24]. These results indicate the importance of long-term follow-up and treatment of severely burned patients.

Post-burn hypermetabolism is initiated to provide sufficient energy for maintaining organ function and whole body homeostasis under demanding trauma conditions [25–28]. Unfortunately, prolonged hypermetabolism becomes detrimental and is associated with vast catabolism, multiorgan failure, and death [1, 29, 30]. Various studies have found that the metabolic need of a burn patient is the highest of any medical state, approaching 140 % of that predicted. The hypermetabolic response involves a vast number of pathways, but there are two, in particular, that appear to most profoundly affect post-burn outcomes: glucose metabolism with insulin resistance (IR) and hyperglycemia [31–34] as well as lipid metabolism with increased lipolysis [35–38].

7.2.1 Glucose Metabolism

During the early post-burn phase, hyperglycemia occurs as a result of an increased rate of glucose appearance, along with an impaired tissue extraction of glucose, leading to an overall increase of glucose and lactate [28, 39]. Of major importance is recent evidence strongly suggesting that hyperglycemia is detrimental and associated with adverse clinical outcomes in severely burned patients. Specifically, studies in burn patients indicated that hyperglycemia is associated with increased infections and sepsis, increased incidence of pneumonia, significantly increased catabolism and hypermetabolism, and, most importantly, with increased post-burn mortality [31–34, 40, 41]. The evidence that hyperglycemia is detrimental in burn patients was further supported by a prospective randomized trial that showed that glucose control is beneficial in terms of post-burn morbidity and organ function [34]. Retrospective cohort studies further confirmed a survival benefit of glucose control in severely burned patients [33, 41]. These data strongly indicate that IR and hyperglycemia represent a significant clinical problem in burn patients and are clearly associated with poor outcome.

Although the dire consequences of burn-induced hyperglycemia have been delineated, the molecular mechanisms underlying IR and hyperglycemia are not entirely defined. Accordingly, ER stress was recently identified as one of the central intracellular stress signaling pathways linking IR, hyperglycemia, and inflammation [42]. Since inflammation, IR, and hyperglycemia are central characteristics of the post-burn response [3], we investigated in a preliminary study whether a severe burn induces ER stress and the unfolded protein response (UPR) in severely burned patients. As expected, we found that a severe thermal injury induces ER stress in the metabolically active tissues skin, fat, and muscle [43]. We therefore have evidence suggesting that ER stress may be central to orchestrating and inducing inflammatory and hypermetabolic responses post-burn on a cellular level.

7.2.2 Fat Metabolism

The other metabolic pathway that is significantly altered during the post-burn hypermetabolic response is lipid metabolism, which may be related to changes in insulin resistance. Lipolysis consists of the breakdown (hydrolysis) of triacylglycerol into free fatty acids (FFA) and glycerol. Notably, lipolysis and free fatty acids not only contribute to post-burn morbidity and mortality by fatty infiltration of various organs, but it was also shown that FFAs can mediate insulin resistance [44]. Specifically, FFAs impair insulin-stimulated glucose uptake [45, 46] and induce insulin resistance through inhibition of glucose transport activity [47]. In the context of type 2 diabetes, it has been shown that increased FFA levels are predictive for incidence and severity of the disease [48]. One of the major alterations post-burn is significantly increased lipolysis, and several studies have suggested that increased lipolysis can be attributed to increased catecholamine levels [49, 50]. Interestingly, despite increased lipolysis, plasma FFA concentrations can be increased or decreased which can be due to hypoalbuminemia or increased intracellular FFA turnover, which is part of the futile cycle involving the breakdown of adipose and muscle TGs into FFA. Regardless, increased triglycerides and FFA lead to fatty infiltration of vital organs, especially the liver. Accordingly, fatty liver is very common post-burn and is associated with increased clinical morbidities, as well as metabolic alterations. Post-burn pathology examinations [51, 52] and spectroscopy studies have shown that burned children have a three to fivefold increase in hepatic triglycerides [53, 54], associated with increased incidence of infection, sepsis, and poor outcome [38]. In addition, hepatic triglyceride levels were higher than those found in diabetic elderly patients, underscoring the metabolic link between fatty infiltration and insulin resistance. This data is in agreement with various other recent studies that showed a strong relationship between fat and glucose metabolism [55]. Though this relationship is clear, the mechanism by which lipids induce insulin resistance is not entirely defined.

7.2.3 Protein Metabolism

Protein/amino acids from skeletal muscle are the major source of fuel in the burned patient, which leads to marked wasting of lean body mass (LBM) within days after injury [1, 56]. Since skeletal muscle has been shown to be responsible for 70–80 % of whole body insulin-stimulated glucose uptake, decreases in muscle mass may significantly contribute to this persistent insulin resistance post-burn [57]. A 10–15 % loss in lean body mass has been shown to be associated with significant increases in infection rate and marked delays in wound healing. The resultant muscle weakness was further shown to prolong mechanical ventilatory requirements, inhibit sufficient cough reflexes, and delay mobilization in protein-malnourished patients, thus markedly contributing to the incidence of mortality in these patients [58]. Persistent protein catabolism may also account for delay in growth frequently observed in our pediatric patient population for up to 2 years post-burn [4].

Various groups suggest that hypermetabolism is a major contributor to poor outcome post-burn and that treatment or alleviation of the hypermetabolic response is beneficial for patient outcomes.

7.3 Attenuation of the Hypermetabolic Response

7.3.1 Non-Pharmacologic Strategies

7.3.1.1 Nutrition

The primary goal of nutritional support is to provide an adequate energy supply and the nutrients necessary to maintain organ function and survival. Early adequate enteral nutrition alleviates catabolism and improves outcomes [59]. However, overfeeding in form of excess calories and/or protein is associated with hyperglycemia, carbon dioxide retention, fatty infiltration of organs, and azotemia [56]. Therefore, nutrition is an essential component to alleviate hypermetabolism, but too much feeding is detrimental and should not be pursued.

Nutritional Route
The preferred route to administer nutrition is oral/NG or NJ tubers. Enteral nutrition (EN) decreases bacteremia, reduces sepsis, maintains motility of the gut, and preserves "first pass" nutrient supply to the liver [59]. In cases where enteral feeding is not applicable (e.g., prolonged ileus or intolerance to enteral feeding), parenteral nutrition should be used to maintain appropriate macro- and micronutrient intake. Parenteral nutrition remains of critical importance in burn patients in whom appropriate dietary support cannot be achieved or in those whose total caloric requirements cannot be fully supplied via enteral nutrition alone.

Initiation of Nutrition
Recently, the initiation of adequate nutrition gained attention and several studies delineated that optimal nutritional support for severely burned patient is best

Table 7.1 Selected enteral nutrition options for burned patients: US market

Nutrition	kcal/ml	CHO g/l (% Cal)	PRO g/l (% Cal)	Fat g/l (% Cal)	Comments
Pediatric					
Vivonex RTF	1	175 (70 %)	50 (20 %)	12 (10 %)	Transitional feeding, low-fat, high-CHO, easily digestible
Vivonex TEN	1	210 (82 %)	38 (15 %)	2.8 (3 %)	Free AA, very low-fat, high-CHO [60]. Severe trauma or surgery
Impact glutamine	1.3	150 (46 %)	78 (24 %)	43 (30 %)	Immunonutrition, GLN, ARG, omega-3 fatty acids
Elecare	0.67	72 (43 %)	20 (15 %)	32 (42 %)	Prepared at 9.4 g/60 ml, AA-based nutrition
Adult					
Crucial	1.5	89 (36 %)	63 (25 %)	45 (39 %)	Immune-enhancing with ARG. Concentrated
Impact	1.0	130 (53 %)	56 (22 %)	28 (25 %)	Immune-enhancing with ARG, GLN, fiber
Oxepa	1.5	105 (28 %)	63 (17 %)	94 (55 %)	ALI, ARDS period (2 week) [61]. Concentrated
Glucerna	1.0	96 (34 %)	42 (17 %)	54 (49 %)	For glucose intolerant or diabetic patients, low CHO
Nepro	1.8	167 (34 %)	81 (18 %)	96 (48 %)	For CKD and patients on dialysis. Concentrated
Osmolite 1 Cal	1.06	144 (54 %)	44 (17 %)	35 (29 %)	Isotonic, for use in intolerance to hyperosmolar nutrition
Modular (children/adult)					
Benefiber powder	0.27	66 (100 %)			(Prepared at 4 g/60 ml) tasteless, odorless, soluble fiber
Beneprotein	0.83		200 (100 %)		(Prepared at 7 g /30 ml) whey protein, mixed in foods

Data extrapolated from "Enteral product Reference Guide, by Nestle Clinical Nutrition 2010" Minneapolis, MN; and "Abbott Nutrition Pocket Guide © 2010"

CHO carbohydrate, *PRO* protein, *AA* amino acid, *GLN* glutamine, *ARG* arginine, *ALI* acute lung injury, *ARDS* acute respiratory distress syndrome, *CKD* chronic kidney disease

accomplished by early (within 12 h after injury) initiation [62]. Beside clinical data, there are animal studies showing that early initiation of enteral nutrition can significantly attenuate the post-burn hypermetabolic responses to severe burn outlined above [59]. Patients with severe burn injury can be safely enterally fed in the duodenum or jejunum within 6 h post-burn, whether or not they have total gastroduodenal function [63]. Thus, nasojejunal or nasoduodenal feeding should be administered early.

Amount of Nutrition

As aforementioned, under- as well as overfeeding is associated with adverse outcomes. Currently, resting energy requirements of burned patients are commonly estimated using equations that incorporate body mass, age, and gender. The performance of these equations has been compared to actual measured resting energy expenditure, which is obtained through indirect calorimetry.

Validation and agreement analysis of formulas such as the Harris-Benedict, Schofield HW, Curreri, and World Health Organization formulas have shown that, although these formulas are based on patient-specific factors such as age, gender, weight, and burn size, they may significantly overestimate caloric requirements in burn patients, increasing the risk of overfeeding and its subsequent deleterious effects [64, 65]. Recently, the adapted Toronto equation seems to be a better formula to calculate REE, as the calculated results very closely matched the MREEs.

We therefore recommend to measure resting energy expenditure via indirect calorimetry and adjust nutrition to this estimation. A factor of 1.2–1.4 is applied to the results of these formulas accounting for the burn hypermetabolic response.

Composition of Nutrition (Table 7.1)

At the moment, no ideal nutrition for burn patients exists. There are only recommendations, and we at RTBC recommend the use of a high glucose, high protein/amino acid, and low-fat nutrition with some unsaturated fatty acids.

We believe that the major energy source for burn patients should be carbohydrates and amino acids thereby sparing protein from oxidation for energy, allowing the protein to be effectively used by the skin and organs. It is estimated that critically ill, burned patients have caloric requirements that far exceed the body's ability to assimilate glucose, which has been reported to be 5 mg/kg/min or approximately 7 g/kg/day (2,240 kcal for an 80 kg man) [66, 67]. However, providing a limited amount of dietary fat diminishes the need for carbohydrates and ameliorates glucose tolerance.

Although the hypermetabolic response to severe burns stimulates lipolysis, the extent to which lipids can be utilized for energy is limited. Thus, fat should comprise less than 25 % of nonprotein calories [68]. Recently, several studies were conducted on the composition of administered fat which showed that the composition of fat is more important than the quantity. Most common lipid sources contain omega-6 polyunsaturated fatty acids such as linoleic acid, which are metabolized to arachidonic acid, a precursor of proinflammatory molecules such as prostaglandin E2 [2, 66]. Omega-3 fatty acids are metabolized without producing proinflammatory compounds. Diets high in omega-3 fatty acids have been associated with an improved inflammatory response, improved outcomes, and reduced incidences of hyperglycemia [69].

Proteolysis is another hallmark of the hypermetabolic response after severe burn injury, and protein loss can exceed 150 g/day [56]. Increased protein catabolism leads to compromised organ function, decreased wound healing, immunoincompetence, and loss of LBM [56]. Evidence suggests that providing a larger protein replacement pool is helpful after severe burn injury [70, 71]. While research has shown that healthy individuals require approximately 1 g/kg/day of protein intake [27, 72–74], in vivo kinetic studies on oxidation rates of amino acids have shown that utilization rates in burned patients are at least 50 % higher than those in healthy, fasting individuals [70, 71]. Thus, at least 1.5–2.0 g/kg/day protein should be given to burn patients. However, supplementation with higher amounts of protein needs to be evaluated carefully as they may fail to yield improvements in muscle protein synthesis or LBM and may serve only to elevate urea production.

Amino acids supplementation was and is controversially discussed, especially alanine and glutamine. Both are important transport amino acids to supply energy to the liver and skin to increase healing mechanisms and metabolic needs [27, 75, 76].

Glutamine also serves as a primary fuel for enterocytes and lymphocytes maintaining small bowel integrity, preserving gut-associated immune function, and limiting intestinal permeability following acute injury [77, 78]. Glutamine is quickly depleted post-burn from serum and muscle [77, 78]; however, this depletion mainly occurs intracellularly, and it is very difficult to deliver glutamine effectively to the cells. Small studies in burn patients indicated that glutamine supplementation decreased incidence of infection, length of stay, and mortality [77, 78]. Therefore, there is a signal that glutamine supplemental maybe associated with beneficial effects. A current multicenter trial (REDOX) is addressing the answer, and the results are expected over the next 4–5 years. The literature on *alanine* is even sparser, and at this time, there is no evidence to administer or not administer alanine. Furthermore, there are no signals whether or not to supplement branched-chain amino acids which improve nitrogen balance [79].

Other important components affected by burns are *vitamins, micronutrients, and trace elements* [80] Table 7.2. Decreased levels of vitamins A, C, D, E, iron, copper, zinc, and selenium have been implicated in wound healing deficiencies and immune dysfunction after severe burn injury [80, 81]. Vitamin A replacement is particularly important for wound healing and epithelial growth. Vitamin C is paramount for the synthesis and cross-linking of collagen post-burn, and burn patients often require up to 20 times the recommended daily allowance [81, 82]. Vitamin D levels are low in burned children, and adequate vitamin D status is likely essential for attenuating further loss of bone minerals post-burn [81, 82].

Trace elements, primarily iron, zinc, selenium, and copper, are required for humoral and cellular immunity [83–89]. Iron is also an important cofactor in oxygen-carrying proteins [56]. Zinc supplementation aids in wound healing, DNA replication, lymphocyte function, and protein synthesis [83–89]. Selenium replacement improves cell-mediated immunity and activates the transcription factor NFkB, a significant modulator of the inflammatory response [83–89]. Copper is critical for collagen synthesis and wound healing [84]. Deficiencies in copper, in particular, have been linked to fatal arrhythmias and poor outcomes [83–89]. Plasma levels of these trace elements are significantly depressed for prolonged periods after the acute burn injury due to increased urinary excretion and significant cutaneous losses. Replacement of these micronutrients lessens morbidity in severely burned patients [83–89]. Therefore, a complete daily multivitamin/mineral supplementation should be given (Table 7.2).

7.3.1.2 Early Excision

Early excision and closure of the burn wound has been probably the single greatest advancement in treating patients with severe thermal injuries during the last two decades leading to substantially reduced resting energy requirements, subsequent improvement of mortality rates, and substantially lower costs in this particular patient population [1, 90, 91]. It is in our opinion imperative to excise the burn wounds early and cover the excised areas with temporary cover materials or autologous skin. This will decrease the burn-induced inflammatory and stress responses leading to decreased hypermetabolism (Fig. 7.2).

7.3.1.3 Environmental Support

Burn patients can lose as much as 4,000 ml/m² burned/day of body water through evaporative loss from extensive burn wounds that have not definitive healed [92]. The altered physiologic state resulting from the hypermetabolic response attempts to at least partly generate sufficient energy to offset heat losses associated with this inevitable water loss. The body attempts to raise skin and core temperatures to 2 °C greater than normal. Raising the ambient temperature from 25 to 33 °C can diminish the magnitude of this obligatory response from 2.0 to 1.4 times the resting energy expenditure in patients exceeding 40 % TBSA. This simple environmental modulation, meaning raise in room temperature, is an important primary treatment goal that frequently is not realized [93] (Fig. 7.2).

7.3.1.4 Exercise and Adjunctive Measures

A balanced physical therapy program is a crucial yet easy intervention to restore metabolic variables and prevent burn-wound contracture. Progressive resistance exercises in convalescent burn patients can maintain and improve body mass, augment incorporation of amino acids into muscle proteins, and increase muscle strength and endurance [64, 94]. It has been demonstrated that resistance exercising can be safely accomplished in pediatric burn patients without exercise-related hyperpyrexia as the result of an inability to dissipate the generated heat [64, 94] (Fig. 7.2).

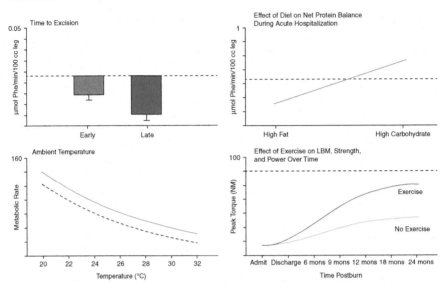

Fig. 7.2 Non-pharmacologic interventions to alleviate hypermetabolism. From Williams FN JACS 2009 April 208(4):489–502

7.3.2 Pharmacologic Modalities

7.3.2.1 Recombinant Human Growth Hormone

Daily intramuscular administration of recombinant human growth hormone (rhGH) at doses of 0.1–0.2 mg/kg as a daily injection during acute burn care has alleviated inflammatory and stress responses [95, 96], increased insulin-like growth factor-I (IGF-I) [97], increased muscle protein kinetics and maintained muscular growth [98, 99], decreased donor site healing time and quality of wound healing [90], improved resting energy expenditure, and decreased cardiac output [100]. However, in a prospective, multicenter, double-blind, randomized, placebo-controlled trial involving 247 patients and 285 critically ill non-burned patients Takala and others found that high doses of rhGH (0.10 ± 0.02 mg/kg BW) were associated with increased morbidity and mortality [101]. Others demonstrated growth hormone treatment to be associated with hyperglycemia and insulin resistance [102, 103]. However, neither short nor long-term administration of rhGH was associated with an increase in mortality in severely burned children [9, 104].

7.3.2.2 Insulin-Like Growth Factor

Because IGF-I mediates the effects of GH, the infusion of equimolar doses of recombinant human IGF-1 and IGFBP-3 as a complex called IGF-I/BP-3 to burned patients improved protein metabolism in catabolic pediatric subjects and adults with significantly less hypoglycemia than rhGH itself [105]. IGF-I/BP-3 attenuates muscle catabolism and improves gut mucosal integrity, improves immune function, attenuate acute phase responses, increased serum concentrations of constitutive proteins, and decreased inflammatory responses [105–108]. However, unpublished data showed that the complex of IGF-I/BP-3 increased neuropathies in severely burned

Table 7.2 Dietary Reference Intakes (DRIs): vitamin and trace elements requirements

Age	Vit A (IU)	Vit D (IU)	Vit E (IU)	Vit C (mg)	Vit K (mcg)	Folate (mcg)	Cu (mg)	Fe (mg)	Se (mcg)	Zn (mg)
0–13 years										
Non-burned	1,300–2,000	200	6–16	15–50	2–60	65–300	0.2–0.7	0.3–8	15–40	2–8
Burned	2,500–5,000			250–500		1,000[a]	0.8–2.8		60–140	12.5–25
≥ 13 years (includes adults)										
Non-burned	2,000–3,000	200–600	23	75–90	75–120	300–400	0.9	8–18	40–60	8–11
Burned	10,000			1,000		1,000[a]	4.0		300–500	25–40

Sources: Dietary reference intakes for calcium, phosphorous, magnesium, vitamin D, and fluoride (1977); dietary reference intakes for thiamin, riboflavin, niacin, vitamin B6, folate, vitamin B12, pantothenic acid, biotin, and choline (1988); dietary reference intakes for vitamin C, vitamin E, selenium, and carotenoids (2000); and dietary reference intakes for vitamin A, vitamin K, arsenic, boron, chromium, copper, iodine, manganese, molybdenum, nickel, silicon, vanadium, and zinc (2001). These reports may be accessed at http://www.nap.edu

Reference Daily Intake (RDI) refers to the daily intake level that a healthy person should achieve. Conversion based on 1 mcg of vit A=3.33 IU of vit A, 1 mcg of calciferol=40 IU of vit D, and 1 mg of α-tocopherol=1.5 IU of vit E

[a]Administered Monday, Wednesday, and Friday

patients and is therefore on hold for clinical use at this moment. Various studies by other investigators indicate the use of IGF-1 alone is not effective in critically ill patients without burns.

7.3.2.3 Oxandrolone

Treatment with anabolic agents such as oxandrolone, a testosterone analog which possesses only 5 % of its virilizing androgenic effects, improves muscle protein catabolism via an increase in protein synthesis [109], reduce weight loss, and increases donor site wound healing [68]. In a prospective randomized study, Wolf and colleagues demonstrated that administration of 10 mg of oxandrolone BiD decreased hospital stay and affected morbidity and mortality [110]. In a large prospective, double-blinded, randomized single-center study, oxandrolone given at a dose of 0.1 mg/kg BiD shortened length of acute hospital stay, maintained LBM and improved body composition and hepatic protein synthesis [111]. The effects were independent of age [112, 113]. Long-term treatment with oxandrolone decreased elevated hypermetabolism and significantly increases body mass over time; lean body mass at 6, 9, and 12 months after burn; and bone mineral content by 12 months after injury versus unburned controls [114, 115]. Patients treated with oxandrolone show few complications, but it should be noted that oxandrolone can increase hepatic enzymes indicating liver damage, especially during acute hospitalization. We recommend checking liver enzymes and markers regularly and in case of hepatic enzyme elevation to stop oxandrolone immediately. In addition, there are reports of oxandrolone causing increased pulmonary fibrosis. If there is any suspicion of pulmonary problems, oxandrolone needs to be stopped.

The dose for adults is 0.1 mg/kg BiD, elderly 0.05 mg/kg BiD.

7.3.2.4 Propranolol

Beta-adrenergic blockade with propranolol represents probably the most efficacious anti-catabolic therapy in the treatment of burns. Acute administration of propranolol exerts anti-inflammatory and antistress effects. Propranolol reduces skeletal muscle wasting and increases lean body mass post-burn [116, 117] and improves glucose metabolism by reducing insulin resistance. Long-term use of propranolol during acute care in burn patients, at a dose titrated to reduce heart rate by 15–20 %, was noted to diminish cardiac work [118]. It also reduced fatty infiltration of the liver, which typically occurs in these patients as the result of enhanced peripheral lipolysis and altered substrate handling. Reduction of hepatic fat results from decreased peripheral lipolysis and reduced palmitate delivery and uptake by the liver [38, 119].

The dose for children is 1 mg/kg given q6 h.

The dose for adults is 10 mg TiD and increases if needed to decrease heart rate to <100 BpM.

7.3.2.5 Insulin

Insulin is a fascinating hormone because of its multifactorial effects. Besides its ability to alter glucose metabolism, insulin has effects on fat and amino acid metabolism and is anabolic.

Stress-induced diabetes with hyperglycemia and insulin resistance during acute hospitalization is a hallmark of severely burned patients and a common pathophysiological phenomenon [3]. During the early phases post-burn, hyperglycemia occurs as a result of an increased rate of glucose appearance along with an impaired tissue extraction of glucose, leading to an increase of glucose and lactate [28, 39]. This pathophysiological post-burn response is similar to the pathophysiology of type 2 diabetes, differing only in its acute onset and severity. Stress-induced hyperglycemia is associated with adverse clinical outcomes after severe burn [31, 32]. Burned patients with poor glucose control have a significantly higher incidence of bacteremia/fungemia and mortality compared to burn patients who have adequate glucose control [31, 32]. We also found that hyperglycemia exaggerates protein degradation, enhancing the catabolic response [31, 32]. Stress-induced diabetes with its insulin resistance and hyperglycemia can be overcome by exogenous insulin administration, which normalizes glucose levels and improves muscle protein synthesis, accelerates donor site healing time, and attenuates lean body mass loss and the acute phase response [12, 120–126]. These data indicate that hyperglycemia associated with insulin resistance represents a significant clinical problem in burn patients and that insulin administration improves morbidity and mortality.

Intensive insulin administration in severely burned patients is associated with beneficial clinical outcomes [12, 41, 120–126]. Intensive insulin therapy to maintain tight euglycemic control, however, represents a difficult clinical effort which has been associated with hypoglycemic episodes. Therefore, the use of a continuous hyperinsulinemic, euglycemic clamp throughout ICU stay has been questioned in multiple multicenter trials throughout the world and has resulted in a dramatic increase in serious hypoglycemic episodes [127]. In a recent multicenter trial in Europe (Efficacy of Volume Substitution and Insulin Therapy in Severe Sepsis (VISEP)), the effect of insulin administration on morbidity and mortality in patients with severe infections and sepsis was investigated [128]. The authors found that insulin administration did not affect mortality, but the rate of severe hypoglycemia was four-fold higher in the intensive therapy group when compared to the conventional therapy group [128]. Maintaining a continuous hyperinsulinemic, euglycemic clamp in burn patients is particularly difficult because these patients are being continuously fed large caloric loads through enteral feeding tubes in an attempt to maintain euglycemia. As burn patients require weekly operations and daily dressing changes, the enteral nutrition occasionally has to be stopped, which lead to disruption of gastrointestinal motility and the risk of hypoglycemia.

We conducted a study to determine the ideal glucose target in severely burned children. We found that 130 mg/dl is the best glucose target, because of glucose levels below 150–160 mg/dl but avoiding detrimental hypoglycemia. Therefore, we recommend at the current time to implement glucose control to a target of 130 mg/dl using insulin.

7.3.2.6 Metformin

Metformin (Glucophage), a biguanide, has recently been suggested as an alternative means to correct hyperglycemia in severely injured patients [129]. By inhibiting gluconeogenesis and augmenting peripheral insulin sensitivity, metformin directly counters the two main metabolic processes which underlie injury-induced hyperglycemia [130, 131]. In addition, metformin has been rarely associated with hypoglycemic events, thus possibly eliminating this concern associated with the use of exogenous insulin [130, 132–134]. In a small randomized study reported by Gore and colleagues, metformin reduced plasma glucose concentration, decreased endogenous glucose production, and accelerated glucose clearance in severely burned [129]. A follow-up study looking at the effects of metformin on muscle protein synthesis confirmed these observations and demonstrated an increased fractional synthetic rate of muscle protein and improvement in net muscle protein balance in metformin-treated patients [130]. Despite the advantages and potential therapeutic uses, treatment with metformin, or other biguanides, has been associated with lactic acidosis [135]. To avoid metformin-associated lactic acidosis, the use of this medication is contraindicated in certain diseases or illnesses in which there is a potential for impaired lactate elimination (hepatic or renal failure) or tissue hypoxia and should be used with caution in subacute burn patients.

Dosing of metformin is 500–1,000 mg BiD p.o.

7.3.2.7 Other Options

Other ongoing trials in order to decrease post-burn hyperglycemia include the use of glucagon-like-peptide (GLP)-1 and PPAR-γ agonists (e.g., pioglitazone, thioglitazones) or the combination of various antidiabetic drugs. PPAR-γ agonists, such as fenofibrate, have been shown to improve insulin sensitivity in patients with diabetes. Cree and colleagues found in a recent double-blind, prospective, placebo-controlled randomized trial that fenofibrate treatment significantly decreased plasma glucose concentrations by improving insulin sensitivity and mitochondrial glucose oxidation [53]. Fenofibrate also led to significantly increased tyrosine phosphorylation of the insulin receptor (IR) and IRS-1 in muscle tissue after hyperinsulinemic-euglycemic clamp when compared to placebo treated patients, indicating improved insulin receptor signaling [53]. GLP-1 has been shown to decrease glucose in severely burned patients, but it was also shown that GLP-1 may not be sufficient to decrease glucose by itself, and insulin needs to be given as an adjunct.

7.4   Summary and Conclusion

The profound metabolic alterations post-burn associated with persistent changes in glucose metabolism and impaired insulin sensitivity significantly contribute to adverse outcome of this patient population. Even though advances in therapy strategies in order to attenuate the hypermetabolic response to burn have significantly improved the clinical outcome of these patients over the past years, therapeutic approaches to overcome this persistent hypermetabolism and associated hyperglycemia have remained challenging. Early excision and closure of the burn wound has been probably the single greatest advancement in the treating patients with severe thermal injuries during the last 20 years, leading to substantially reduced resting energy requirements and subsequent improvement of mortality rates in this particular patient population. At present, beta-adrenergic blockade with propranolol represents probably the most efficacious anti-catabolic therapy in the treatment of burns. Other pharmacological strategies that have been successfully utilized in order to attenuate the hypermetabolic response to burn injury include growth hormone, insulin-like growth factor, and oxandrolone. Maintaining blood glucose at levels below 130 mg/dl using intensive insulin therapy has been shown to reduce mortality and morbidity in critically ill patients: however, associated hypoglycemic events have led to the investigation of alternative strategies, including the use of metformin and the PPAR-γ agonist fenofibrate. Nevertheless, further studies are warranted to determine ideal glucose ranges and the safety and the appropriate use of the above-mentioned drugs in critically ill patients.

References

1. Herndon DN, Tompkins RG (2004) Support of the metabolic response to burn injury. Lancet 363:1895–1902
2. Kraft R, Herndon DN, Al-Mousawi AM, Williams FN, Finnerty CC, Jeschke MG (2012) Burn size and survival probability in paediatric patients in modern burn care: a prospective observational cohort study. Lancet 379:1013–1021
3. Jeschke MG, Chinkes DL, Finnerty CC et al (2008) Pathophysiologic response to severe burn injury. Ann Surg 248:387–401
4. Jeschke MG, Gauglitz GG, Kulp GA et al (2011) Long-term persistance of the pathophysiologic response to severe burn injury. PLoS One 6:e21245
5. McCowen KC, Malhotra A, Bistrian BR (2001) Stress-induced hyperglycemia. Crit Care Clin 17:107–124
6. Hart DW, Wolf SE, Chinkes DL et al (2000) Determinants of skeletal muscle catabolism after severe burn. Ann Surg 232:455–465
7. Mlcak RP, Jeschke MG, Barrow RE, Herndon DN (2006) The influence of age and gender on resting energy expenditure in severely burned children. Ann Surg 244:121–130
8. Przkora R, Barrow RE, Jeschke MG et al (2006) Body composition changes with time in pediatric burn patients. J Trauma 60:968–971; discussion 71
9. Przkora R, Herndon DN, Suman OE et al (2006) Beneficial effects of extended growth hormone treatment after hospital discharge in pediatric burn patients. Ann Surg 243:796–801; discussion 3
10. Dolecek R (1989) Endocrine changes after burn trauma – a review. Keio J Med 38:262–276
11. Jeffries MK, Vance ML (1992) Growth hormone and cortisol secretion in patients with burn injury. J Burn Care Rehabil 13:391–395
12. Jeschke MG, Klein D, Herndon DN (2004) Insulin treatment improves the systemic inflammatory reaction to severe trauma. Ann Surg 239:553–560
13. Goodall M, Stone C, Haynes BW Jr (1957) Urinary output of adrenaline and noradrenaline in severe thermal burns. Ann Surg 145:479–487
14. Coombes EJ, Batstone GF (1982) Urine cortisol levels after burn injury. Burns Incl Therm Inj 8:333–337
15. Norbury WB, Herndon DN (2007) Modulation of the hypermetabolic response after burn injury. In: Herndon DN (ed) Total burn care, 3rd edn. Saunders Elsevier, New York, pp 420–433
16. Sheridan RL (2001) A great constitutional disturbance. N Engl J Med 345:1271–1272
17. Pereira C, Murphy K, Jeschke M, Herndon DN (2005) Post burn muscle wasting and the effects of treatments. Int J Biochem Cell Biol 37:1948–1961

18. Wolfe RR (1981) Review: acute versus chronic response to burn injury. Circ Shock 8:105–115
19. Cuthbertson DP, Angeles Valero Zanuy MA, Leon Sanz ML (2001) Post-shock metabolic response. 1942. Nutr Hosp 16:176–182; discussion 5–6
20. Galster AD, Bier DM, Cryer PE, Monafo WW (1984) Plasma palmitate turnover in subjects with thermal injury. J Trauma 24:938–945
21. Cree MG, Wolfe RR (2008) Postburn trauma insulin resistance and fat metabolism. Am J Physiol Endocrinol Metab 294:E1–E9
22. Childs C, Heath DF, Little RA, Brotherston M (1990) Glucose metabolism in children during the first day after burn injury. Arch Emerg Med 7:135–147
23. Cree MG, Aarsland A, Herndon DN, Wolfe RR (2007) Role of fat metabolism in burn trauma-induced skeletal muscle insulin resistance. Crit Care Med 35:S476–S483
24. Gauglitz GG, Herndon DN, Kulp GA, Meyer WJ 3rd, Jeschke MG (2009) Abnormal insulin sensitivity persists up to three years in pediatric patients post-burn. J Clin Endocrinol Metabol 94:1656–1664
25. Wolfe RR, Durkot MJ, Allsop JR, Burke JF (1979) Glucose metabolism in severely burned patients. Metabolism 28:1031–1039
26. Wolfe RR, Herndon DN, Peters EJ, Jahoor F, Desai MH, Holland OB (1987) Regulation of lipolysis in severely burned children. Ann Surg 206:214–221
27. Wolfe RR, Jahoor F, Hartl WH (1989) Protein and amino acid metabolism after injury. Diabetes Metab Rev 5:149–164
28. Wolfe RR, Miller HI, Spitzer JJ (1977) Glucose and lactate kinetics in burn shock. Am J Physiol 232:E415–E418
29. Wilmore DW (1976) Hormonal responses and their effect on metabolism. Surg Clin North Am 56:999–1018
30. Wilmore DW, Aulick LH (1978) Metabolic changes in burned patients. Surg Clin North Am 58:1173–1187
31. Gore DC, Chinkes D, Heggers J, Herndon DN, Wolf SE, Desai M (2001) Association of hyperglycemia with increased mortality after severe burn injury. J Trauma 51:540–544
32. Gore DC, Chinkes DL, Hart DW, Wolf SE, Herndon DN, Sanford AP (2002) Hyperglycemia exacerbates muscle protein catabolism in burn-injured patients. Crit Care Med 30:2438–2442
33. Hemmila MR, Taddonio MA, Arbabi S, Maggio PM, Wahl WL (2008) Intensive insulin therapy is associated with reduced infectious complications in burn patients. Surgery 144: 629–635; discussion 35–37
34. Jeschke MG, Kulp GA, Kraft R et al (2010) Intensive insulin therapy in severely burned pediatric patients: a prospective randomized trial. Am J Respir Crit Care Med 182:351–359
35. Barrow RE, Wolfe RR, Dasu MR, Barrow LN, Herndon DN (2006) The use of beta-adrenergic blockade in preventing trauma-induced hepatomegaly. Ann Surg 243:115–120
36. Martini WZ, Irtun O, Chinkes DL, Rasmussen B, Traber DL, Wolfe RR (2001) Alteration of hepatic fatty acid metabolism after burn injury in pigs. JPEN J Parenter Enteral Nutr 25:310–316
37. Morio B, Irtun O, Herndon DN, Wolfe RR (2002) Propranolol decreases splanchnic triacylglycerol storage in burn patients receiving a high-carbohydrate diet. Ann Surg 236:218–225
38. Barret JP, Jeschke MG, Herndon DN (2001) Fatty infiltration of the liver in severely burned pediatric patients: autopsy findings and clinical implications. J Trauma 51:736–739
39. Gore DC, Ferrando A, Barnett J et al (2000) Influence of glucose kinetics on plasma lactate concentration and energy expenditure in severely burned patients. J Trauma 49:673–677; discussion 7–8
40. Jeschke MG, Klein D, Thasler WE et al (2008) Insulin decreases inflammatory signal transcription factor expression in primary human liver cells after LPS challenge. Mol Med 14:11–19
41. Pham TN, Warren AJ, Phan HH, Molitor F, Greenhalgh DG, Palmieri TL (2005) Impact of tight glycemic control in severely burned children. J Trauma 59:1148–1154
42. Zhang K, Kaufman RJ (2008) From endoplasmic-reticulum stress to the inflammatory response. Nature 454:455–462

43. Jeschke MG, Finnerty CC, Herndon DN et al (2012) Severe injury is associated with insulin resistance, endoplasmic reticulum stress response, and unfolded protein response. Ann Surg 255:370–378
44. Randle PJ, Garland PB, Hales CN, Newsholme EA (1963) The glucose fatty-acid cycle. Its role in insulin sensitivity and the metabolic disturbances of diabetes mellitus. Lancet 1:785–789
45. Boden G, Chen X, Ruiz J, Heifets M, Morris M, Badosa F (1994) Insulin receptor down-regulation and impaired antilipolytic action of insulin in diabetic patients after pancreas/kidney transplantation. J Clin Endocrinol Metabol 78:657–663
46. Shah P, Vella A, Basu A et al (2002) Effects of free fatty acids and glycerol on splanchnic glucose metabolism and insulin extraction in nondiabetic humans. Diabetes 51:301–310
47. Dresner A, Laurent D, Marcucci M et al (1999) Effects of free fatty acids on glucose transport and IRS-1-associated phosphatidylinositol 3-kinase activity. J Clin Invest 103:253–259
48. Pankow JS, Duncan BB, Schmidt MI et al (2004) Fasting plasma free fatty acids and risk of type 2 diabetes: the atherosclerosis risk in communities study. Diabetes Care 27:77–82
49. Herndon DN, Nguyen TT, Wolfe RR et al (1994) Lipolysis in burned patients is stimulated by the beta 2-receptor for catecholamines. Arch Surg 129:1301–1304; discussion 4–5
50. Wolfe RR, Herndon DN, Jahoor F, Miyoshi H, Wolfe M (1987) Effect of severe burn injury on substrate cycling by glucose and fatty acids. N Engl J Med 317:403–408
51. Barrow RE, Hawkins HK, Aarsland A et al (2005) Identification of factors contributing to hepatomegaly in severely burned children. Shock 24:523–528
52. Jeschke MG (2009) The hepatic response to thermal injury: is the liver important for postburn outcomes? Mol Med 15:337–351
53. Cree MG, Newcomer BR, Herndon DN et al (2007) PPAR-alpha agonism improves whole body and muscle mitochondrial fat oxidation, but does not alter intracellular fat concentrations in burn trauma children in a randomized controlled trial. Nutr Metab (Lond) 4:9
54. Cree MG, Newcomer BR, Katsanos CS et al (2004) Intramuscular and liver triglycerides are increased in the elderly. J Clin Endocrinol Metabol 89:3864–3871
55. Petersen KF, Befroy D, Dufour S et al (2003) Mitochondrial dysfunction in the elderly: possible role in insulin resistance. Science 300:1140–1142
56. Saffle JR, Graves C (2007) Nutritional support of the burned patient. In: Herndon DN (ed) Total burn care, 3rd edn. Saunders Elsevier, London, pp 398–419
57. DeFronzo RA, Jacot E, Jequier E, Maeder E, Wahren J, Felber JP (1981) The effect of insulin on the disposal of intravenous glucose. Results from indirect calorimetry and hepatic and femoral venous catheterization. Diabetes 30:1000–1007
58. Arora NS, Rochester DF (1982) Respiratory muscle strength and maximal voluntary ventilation in undernourished patients. Am Rev Respir Dis 126:5–8
59. Mochizuki H, Trocki O, Dominioni L, Brackett KA, Joffe SN, Alexander JW (1984) Mechanism of prevention of postburn hypermetabolism and catabolism by early enteral feeding. Ann Surg 200:297–310
60. Hart DW, Wolf SE, Zhang XJ et al (2001) Efficacy of a high-carbohydrate diet in catabolic illness. Crit Care Med 29:1318–1324
61. Mayes T, Gottschlich MM, Kagan RJ (2008) An evaluation of the safety and efficacy of an anti-inflammatory, pulmonary enteral formula in the treatment of pediatric burn patients with respiratory failure. J Burn Care Res 29:82–88
62. Gore DC, Chinkes D, Sanford A, Hart DW, Wolf SE, Herndon DN (2003) Influence of fever on the hypermetabolic response in burn-injured children. Arch Surg 138:169–174; discussion 74
63. Raff T, Germann G, Hartmann B (1997) The value of early enteral nutrition in the prophylaxis of stress ulceration in the severely burned patient. Burns 23:313–318
64. Suman OE, Mlcak RP, Chinkes DL, Herndon DN (2006) Resting energy expenditure in severely burned children: analysis of agreement between indirect calorimetry and prediction equations using the Bland-Altman method. Burns 32:335–342
65. Gore DC, Rutan RL, Hildreth M, Desai MH, Herndon DN (1990) Comparison of resting energy expenditures and caloric intake in children with severe burns. J Burn Care Rehabil 11:400–404

66. Wolfe RR (1993) Metabolic response to burn injury: nutritional implications. Semin Nephrol 13:382–390
67. Wolfe RR (1998) Metabolic interactions between glucose and fatty acids in humans. Am J Clin Nutr 67:519S–526S
68. Demling RH, Seigne P (2000) Metabolic management of patients with severe burns. World J Surg 24:673–680
69. Alexander JW, William A (1986) Altemeier lecture. Nutrition and infection. New perspectives for an old problem. Arch Surg 121:966–972
70. Wolfe RR, Shaw JH, Durkot MJ (1983) Energy metabolism in trauma and sepsis: the role of fat. Prog Clin Biol Res 111:89–109
71. Yu B, Wang S, You Z (1995) Enhancement of gut absorptive function by early enteral feeding enriched with L-glutamine in severe burned miniswines. Zhonghua Wai Ke Za Zhi 33:742–744
72. Wolfe RR (1997) Substrate utilization/insulin resistance in sepsis/trauma. Baillieres Clin Endocrinol Metab 11:645–657
73. Wolfe RR, Durkot MJ, Wolfe MH (1982) Effect of thermal injury on energy metabolism, substrate kinetics, and hormonal concentrations. Circ Shock 9:383–394
74. Wolfe RR, Klein S, Herndon DN, Jahoor F (1990) Substrate cycling in thermogenesis and amplification of net substrate flux in human volunteers and burned patients. J Trauma 30:S6–S9
75. Andel H, Kamolz LP, Horauf K, Zimpfer M (2003) Nutrition and anabolic agents in burned patients. Burns 29:592–595
76. Peng X, Chen RC, Wang P, You ZY, Wang SL (2004) Effects of enteral supplementation with glutamine on mitochondria respiratory function of intestinal epithelium in burned rats. Zhongguo Wei Zhong Bing Ji Jiu Yi Xue 16:93–96
77. Wischmeyer PE (2006) The glutamine story: where are we now? Curr Opin Crit Care 12:142–148
78. Wischmeyer PE, Lynch J, Liedel J et al (2001) Glutamine administration reduces gram-negative bacteremia in severely burned patients: a prospective, randomized, double-blind trial versus isonitrogenous control. Crit Care Med 29:2075–2080
79. Cerra FB, Siegel JH, Coleman B, Border JR, McMenamy RR (1980) Septic autocannibalism. A failure of exogenous nutritional support. Ann Surg 192:570–580
80. Gamliel Z, DeBiasse MA, Demling RH (1996) Essential microminerals and their response to burn injury. J Burn Care Rehabil 17:264–272
81. Gottschlich MM, Mayes T, Khoury J, Warden GD (2004) Hypovitaminosis D in acutely injured pediatric burn patients. J Am Diet Assoc 104:931–941, quiz 1031
82. Mayes T, Gottschlich MM, Warden GD (1997) Clinical nutrition protocols for continuous quality improvements in the outcomes of patients with burns. J Burn Care Rehabil 18: 365–368; discussion 4
83. Berger MM, Shenkin A (2007) Trace element requirements in critically ill burned patients. J Trace Elem Med Biol 21(Suppl 1):44–48
84. Berger MM, Binnert C, Chiolero RL et al (2007) Trace element supplementation after major burns increases burned skin trace element concentrations and modulates local protein metabolism but not whole-body substrate metabolism. Am J Clin Nutr 85:1301–1306
85. Berger MM, Baines M, Raffoul W et al (2007) Trace element supplementation after major burns modulates antioxidant status and clinical course by way of increased tissue trace element concentrations. Am J Clin Nutr 85:1293–1300
86. Berger MM, Eggimann P, Heyland DK et al (2006) Reduction of nosocomial pneumonia after major burns by trace element supplementation: aggregation of two randomised trials. Crit Care 10:R153
87. Berger MM (2006) Antioxidant micronutrients in major trauma and burns: evidence and practice. Nutr Clin Pract 21:438–449
88. Berger MM, Shenkin A (2006) Vitamins and trace elements: practical aspects of supplementation. Nutrition 22:952–955

89. Berger MM (2005) Can oxidative damage be treated nutritionally? Clin Nutr 24:172–183
90. Herndon DN, Hawkins HK, Nguyen TT, Pierre E, Cox R, Barrow RE (1995) Characterization of growth hormone enhanced donor site healing in patients with large cutaneous burns. Ann Surg 221:649–656
91. Solomon JR (1981) Early surgical excision and grafting of burns including tangential excision. Prog Pediatr Surg 14:133–149
92. Zawacki BE, Spitzer KW, Mason AD Jr, Johns LA (1970) Does increased evaporative water loss cause hypermetabolism in burned patients? Ann Surg 171:236–240
93. Wilmore DW, Mason AD Jr, Johnson DW, Pruitt BA Jr (1975) Effect of ambient temperature on heat production and heat loss in burn patients. J Appl Physiol 38:593–597
94. Suman OE, Spies RJ, Celis MM, Mlcak RP, Herndon DN (2001) Effects of a 12-week resistance exercise program on skeletal muscle strength in children with burn injuries. J Appl Physiol 91:1168–1175
95. Jeschke MG, Herndon DN, Wolf SE et al (1999) Recombinant human growth hormone alters acute phase reactant proteins, cytokine expression, and liver morphology in burned rats. J Surg Res 83:122–129
96. Wu X, Thomas SJ, Herndon DN, Sanford AP, Wolf SE (2004) Insulin decreases hepatic acute phase protein levels in severely burned children. Surgery 135:196–202
97. Jeschke MG, Chrysopoulo MT, Herndon DN, Wolf SE (1999) Increased expression of insulin-like growth factor-I in serum and liver after recombinant human growth hormone administration in thermally injured rats. J Surg Res 85:171–177
98. Aili Low JF, Barrow RE, Mittendorfer B, Jeschke MG, Chinkes DL, Herndon DN (2001) The effect of short-term growth hormone treatment on growth and energy expenditure in burned children. Burns 27:447–452
99. Hart DW, Wolf SE, Beauford RB, Lal SO, Chinkes DL, Herndon DN (2001) Determinants of blood loss during primary burn excision. Surgery 130:396–402
100. Branski LK, Herndon DN, Barrow RE et al (2009) Randomized controlled trial to determine the efficacy of long-term growth hormone treatment in severely burned children. Ann Surg 250(4):514–523
101. Takala J, Ruokonen E, Webster NR et al (1999) Increased mortality associated with growth hormone treatment in critically ill adults. N Engl J Med 341:785–792
102. Gore DC, Honeycutt D, Jahoor F, Wolfe RR, Herndon DN (1991) Effect of exogenous growth hormone on whole-body and isolated-limb protein kinetics in burned patients. Arch Surg 126:38–43
103. Demling R (1999) Growth hormone therapy in critically ill patients. N Engl J Med 341:837–839
104. Ramirez RJ, Wolf SE, Barrow RE, Herndon DN (1998) Growth hormone treatment in pediatric burns: a safe therapeutic approach. Ann Surg 228:439–448
105. Herndon DN, Ramzy PI, Debroy MA et al (1999) Muscle protein catabolism after severe burn, effects of IGF-1/IGFBP3 treatment. Ann Surg 229:713–720
106. Spies M, Wolf SE, Barrow RE, Jeschke MG, Herndon DN (2002) Modulation of types I and II acute phase reactants with insulin-like growth factor-1/binding protein-3 complex in severely burned children. Crit Care Med 30:83–88
107. Jeschke MG, Barrow RE, Herndon DN (2000) Insulinlike growth factor I plus insulinlike growth factor binding protein 3 attenuates the proinflammatory acute phase response in severely burned children. Ann Surg 231:246–252
108. Cioffi WG, Gore DC, Rue LW III et al (1994) Insulin-like growth factor-1 lowers protein oxidation in patients with thermal injury. Ann Surg 220(3):310–319
109. Hart DW, Wolf SE, Ramzy PI et al (2001) Anabolic effects of oxandrolone after severe burn. Ann Surg 233:556–564
110. Wolf SE, Edelman LS, Kemalyan N et al (2006) Effects of oxandrolone on outcome measures in the severely burned: a multicenter prospective randomized double-blind trial. J Burn Care Res 27:131–141

111. Jeschke MG, Finnerty CC, Suman OE, Kulp G, Mlcak RP, Herndon DN (2007) The effect of oxandrolone on the endocrinologic, inflammatory, and hypermetabolic responses during the acute phase postburn. Ann Surg 246:351–362

112. Demling RH, DeSanti L (2003) Oxandrolone induced lean mass gain during recovery from severe burns is maintained after discontinuation of the anabolic steroid. Burns 29:793–797

113. Demling RH, DeSanti L (2001) The rate of restoration of body weight after burn injury, using the anabolic agent oxandrolone, is not age dependent. Burns 27:46–51

114. Pham TN, Klein MB, Gibran NS et al (2008) Impact of oxandrolone treatment on acute outcomes after severe burn injury. J Burn Care Res 29:902–906

115. Przkora R, Herndon DN, Suman OE (2007) The effects of oxandrolone and exercise on muscle mass and function in children with severe burns. Pediatrics 119:e109–e116

116. Gore DC, Honeycutt D, Jahoor F, Barrow RE, Wolfe RR, Herndon DN (1991) Propranolol diminishes extremity blood flow in burned patients. Ann Surg 213:568–573; discussion 73–74

117. Herndon DN, Hart DW, Wolf SE, Chinkes DL, Wolfe RR (2001) Reversal of catabolism by beta-blockade after severe burns. N Engl J Med 345:1223–1229

118. Baron PW, Barrow RE, Pierre EJ, Herndon DN (1997) Prolonged use of propranolol safely decreases cardiac work in burned children. J Burn Care Rehabil 18:223–227

119. Aarsland A, Chinkes D, Wolfe RR et al (1996) Beta-blockade lowers peripheral lipolysis in burn patients receiving growth hormone. Rate of hepatic very low density lipoprotein triglyceride secretion remains unchanged. Ann Surg 223:777–787; discussion 87–89

120. Ferrando AA, Chinkes DL, Wolf SE, Matin S, Herndon DN, Wolfe RR (1999) A submaximal dose of insulin promotes net skeletal muscle protein synthesis in patients with severe burns. Ann Surg 229:11–18

121. Pierre EJ, Barrow RE, Hawkins HK et al (1998) Effects of insulin on wound healing. J Trauma 44:342–345

122. Thomas SJ, Morimoto K, Herndon DN et al (2002) The effect of prolonged euglycemic hyperinsulinemia on lean body mass after severe burn. Surgery 132:341–347

123. Zhang XJ, Chinkes DL, Wolf SE, Wolfe RR (1999) Insulin but not growth hormone stimulates protein anabolism in skin would and muscle. Am J Physiol 276:E712–E720

124. Jeschke MG, Klein D, Bolder U, Einspanier R (2004) Insulin attenuates the systemic inflammatory response in endotoxemic rats. Endocrinology 145:4084–4093

125. Jeschke MG, Rensing H, Klein D et al (2005) Insulin prevents liver damage and preserves liver function in lipopolysaccharide-induced endotoxemic rats. J Hepatol 42:870–879

126. Klein D, Schubert T, Horch RE, Jauch KW, Jeschke MG (2004) Insulin treatment improves hepatic morphology and function through modulation of hepatic signals after severe trauma. Ann Surg 240:340–349

127. Langouche L, Vanhorebeek I, Van den Berghe G (2007) Therapy insight: the effect of tight glycemic control in acute illness. Nat Clin Pract Endocrinol Metab 3:270–278

128. Brunkhorst FM, Engel C, Bloos F et al (2008) Intensive insulin therapy and pentastarch resuscitation in severe sepsis. N Engl J Med 358:125–139

129. Gore DC, Wolf SE, Herndon DN, Wolfe RR (2003) Metformin blunts stress-induced hyperglycemia after thermal injury. J Trauma 54:555–561

130. Gore DC, Wolf SE, Sanford A, Herndon DN, Wolfe RR (2005) Influence of metformin on glucose intolerance and muscle catabolism following severe burn injury. Ann Surg 241:334–342

131. Moon RJ, Bascombe LA, Holt RI (2007) The addition of metformin in type 1 diabetes improves insulin sensitivity, diabetic control, body composition and patient well-being. Diabetes Obes Metab 9:143–145

132. Staels B (2006) Metformin and pioglitazone: effectively treating insulin resistance. Curr Med Res Opin 22(Suppl 2):S27–S37

133. Musi N, Goodyear LJ (2006) Insulin resistance and improvements in signal transduction. Endocrine 29:73–80

134. Hundal RS, Inzucchi SE (2003) Metformin: new understandings, new uses. Drugs 63: 1879–1894

135. Tahrani AA, Varughese GI, Scarpello JH, Hanna FW (2007) Metformin, heart failure, and lactic acidosis: is metformin absolutely contraindicated? BMJ 335:508–512

Nursing Management of the Burn-Injured Person

8

Judy Knighton

8.1 Introduction

The repertoire of skills needed to provide care to the burn-injured patient includes comprehensive clinical assessment and monitoring, pain management, wound care and psychosocial support. This chapter is focused on providing the nurse with valuable information for the provision of appropriate nursing care.

8.2 Knowledge Base

8.2.1 General Definition and Description

8.2.1.1 Incidence

- Annually, an estimated 450,000 people seek care for burns in the USA [1, 2].
- Approximately 45,000 require hospitalisation, greater than half of whom (25,000) receive care in specialised burn units or centres [1, 2].
- Survival rate, for hospitalised patients, is around 96 %.
- Children 4 years of age and younger and adults over the age of 55 form the largest group of fatalities.
- In North America and Europe, 70 % of burn survivors are male and 30 % female.

J. Knighton, RN, MScN
Ross Tilley Burn Centre, Sunnybrook Health Sciences Centre,
2075 Bayview Ave. D7-14, Toronto, ON, M4N 3M5, Canada
e-mail: judy.knighton@sunnybrook.ca

M.G. Jeschke et al. (eds.), *Burn Care and Treatment*,
DOI 10.1007/978-3-7091-1133-8_8, © Springer-Verlag Wien 2013

Table 8.1 American Burn Association adult burn classification

Classification	Assessment criteria
Minor burn injury	<15 % TBSA burn in adults <40 years age
	<10 % TBSA burn in adults >40 years age
	<2 % TBSA full-thickness burn without risk of functional or aesthetic impairment or disability
Moderate uncomplicated burn injury	15–25 % TBSA burn in adults <40 years age
	10–20 % TBSA burn in adults >40 years age
	<10 % TBSA full-thickness burn without functional or aesthetic risk to burns involving the face, eyes, ears, hands, feet or perineum
Major burn injury	>25 % TBSA burn in adults <40 years age
	>20 % TBSA burn in adults >40 years age
	OR >10 % TBSA full-thickness burn (any age)
	OR injuries involving the face, eyes, ears, hands, feet
	OR perineum likely to result in functional or aesthetic disability
	OR high-voltage electrical burn
	OR all burns with inhalation injury or major trauma

8.2.1.2 Classification

Burn complexity can range from a relatively minor, uncomplicated injury to a life-threatening, multisystem trauma. The American Burn Association (ABA) has a useful classification system that rates burn injury magnitude from minor to moderate, uncomplicated to major (Table 8.1).

8.3 Aetiology and Risk Factors

The causes of burn injuries are numerous and found in both the home, leisure and workplace settings (Table 8.2).

8.3.1 Pathophysiology

8.3.1.1 Severity Factors

There are five factors that need to be considered when determining the severity of a burn injury (Box 8.1):

1. *Extent* – There are several methods available to accurately calculate the percentage of body surface area involved:
   - The simplest is the rule of nines (see Chap. 1, Fig. 1.1 and Chap. 2, Fig. 2.2). *However, it is only for use with the adult burn population.*
   - The Lund and Browder method (see Chap. 1, Fig. 1.1 and Chap. 2, Fig. 2.2) is useful for all age groups, but is more complicated to use.
   - There is a paediatric version of the Lund and Browder method (see Chap. 2, Fig. 2.2).

Table 8.2 Causes of burn injuries

Home and leisure	Workplace
Hot water heaters set too high (140 °F or 60 °C)	Electricity:
Overloaded electrical outlets	Power lines
Frayed electrical wiring	Outlet boxes
Carelessness with cigarettes, lighters, matches, candles	Chemicals:
Pressure cookers	Acids
Microwaved foods and liquids	Alkalis
Hot grease or cooking liquids	Tar
Open space heaters	Hot steam sources:
Gas fireplace doors	Boilers
Radiators	Pipes
Hot sauna rocks	Industrial cookers
Improper use of flammable liquids:	Hot industrial presses
Starter fluids	Flammable liquids:
Gasoline	Propane
Kerosene	Acetylene
Electrical storms	Natural gas
Overexposure to sun	

Box 8.1. Burn Severity Factors
1. Extent of body surface area burned
2. Depth of tissue damage
3. Age of person
4. Part of body burned
5. Past medical history

- If the burned areas are scattered, small and irregularly shaped, the rule of palm can be used. The palm of the burned person's hand represents 1 % body surface area.
- If 10 % or more of the body surface of a child or 15 % or more of that of an adult is burned, the injury is considered serious. The person requires hospitalisation and fluid replacement to prevent shock.

2. Depth
   - Two factors determine the depth of a burn wound: temperature of the burning agent and duration of exposure time.
   - Previous terminology to describe burn depth was first, second and third degree. In recent years, these terms have been replaced by those more descriptive in nature: superficial partial-thickness, deep partial-thickness and full-thickness (Table 8.3).
   - Superficial burns, such as those produced by sunburn, are not taken into consideration when assessing extent and depth.

Table 8.3 Classification of burn injury depth

Degree of burn	Cause of injury	Depth of injury	Appearance	Treatment
First degree	Superficial sunburn Brief exposure to hot liquids or heat flash	Superficial damage to epithelium Tactile and pain sensations intact	Erythematous, blanching on pressure, no blisters	Complete healing within 3–5 days with no scarring
Superficial partial-thickness (second degree)	Brief exposure to flame, flash or hot liquids	Destruction of epidermis, superficial damage to upper layer of dermis, epidermal appendages intact	Moist, weepy, blanching on pressure, blisters, pink or red colour	Complete healing within 14–21 days with no scarring
Deep partial-thickness (deep second degree)	Exposure to flame, scalding liquids or hot tar	Destruction of epidermis, damage to dermis, some epidermal appendages intact	Pale and less moist, no blanching or prolonged, deep pressure sensation intact, pinprick sensation absent	Prolonged healing time usually >21 days with scarring. Skin grafting may be necessary for improved functional and aesthetic outcome
Full-thickness (third degree)	Prolonged contact with flame, steam, scalding liquids, hot objects, chemicals or electrical current	Complete destruction of epidermis, dermis and epidermal appendages; injury through most of the dermis	Dry, leathery, pale, mottled brown or red in colour; visible thrombosed vessels insensitive to pain and pressure	Requires skin grafting
Full-thickness (fourth degree)	Major electrical current, prolonged contact with heat source (i.e. unconscious patient)	Complete destruction of epidermis, dermis and epidermal appendages; injury involving connective tissue, muscle and bone	Dry, black, mottled brown, white or red; no sensation and limited movement of burned limbs or digits	Requires skin grafting and likely amputation

- The skin is divided into three layers, which include the epidermis, dermis and subcutaneous tissue (Fig. 8.1).
3. Age
   - For patients less than 2 years of age and greater than 50, there is a higher incidence of morbidity and mortality.
   - Sadly, the infant, toddler and elderly are at increased risk for abuse by burning.
4. Part of the body burned
   - Patients with burns to the face, neck, hands, feet or perineum have greater challenges to overcome and require the specialised care offered by a burn centre.
5. Past medical history
   - Pre-existing cardiovascular, pulmonary or renal disease will be exacerbated by the burn injury.
   - Persons with diabetes or peripheral vascular disease have a more difficult time with wound healing, especially on the legs and feet.

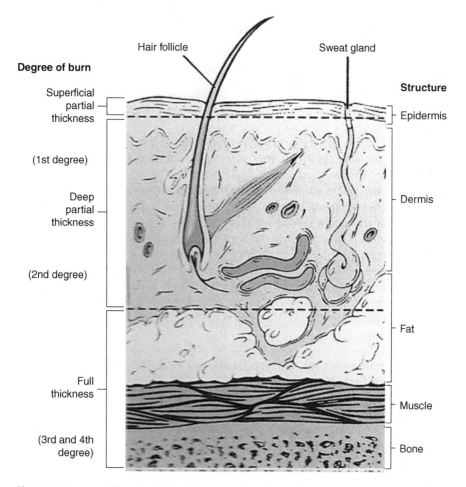

Fig. 8.1 Anatomy of burn tissue depth

8.3.2 Local Damage

Local damage varies, depending upon:
(a) Temperature of the burning agent
(b) Duration of contact time
(c) Type of tissue involved
Zones of tissue damage:
- Inner zone of *coagulation* (full-thickness injury) – irreversible cell death, skin grafting needed for permanent coverage
- Middle zone of *stasis* (deep, partial-thickness injury) – some skin-reproducing cells present in the dermal appendages with circulation partially intact, healing generally within 14–21 days
- Outer zone of *hyperaemia* (superficial, partial-thickness injury) – minimal cell involvement and spontaneous healing within 7–10 days

8.3.3 Fluid and Electrolyte Shifts

The immediate post-burn period is marked by dramatic circulation changes, producing what is known as "burn shock" (Fig. 8.2).
- As the capillary walls begin leaking, water, sodium and plasma proteins (primarily albumin) move into the interstitial spaces in a phenomenon known as "second spacing".
- When the fluid begins to accumulate in areas where there is normally minimal to no fluid, the term "third spacing" is used. This fluid is found in exudate and blisters.
- There is also insensible fluid loss through evaporation from large, open body surfaces. A non-burned individual loses about 30–50 mL/h. A severely burned patient may lose anywhere from 200 to 400 mL/h.
- Circulation is also impaired in the burn patient due to haemolysis of red blood cells.
- Following successful completion of the fluid resuscitation phase, capillary membrane permeability is restored. Fluids gradually shift back from the interstitial space to the intravascular space, and the patient is no longer grossly oedematous and diuresis is ongoing.

8.4 Cardiovascular, Gastrointestinal and Renal System Manifestations

During the hypovolemic shock phase, only vital areas of circulation are maintained.
- Cardiac monitoring is essential, particularly if the patient has a pre-burn history of cardiac problems.
- Electrical burn patients, who arrest at the scene or who experience cardiac arrhythmias post-injury, warrant particular vigilance.

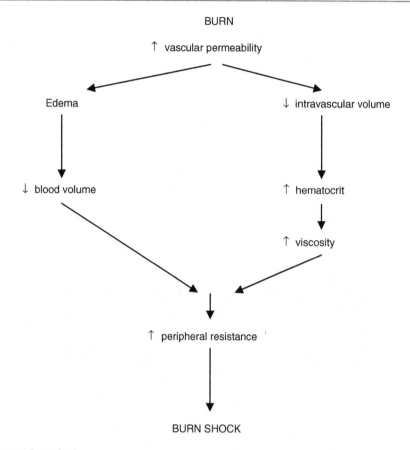

Fig. 8.2 Burn shock

- Hypovolemic shock and hypoxemia also produce the initial gastrointestinal complications seen post-burn, such as decreased peristalsis and abdominal paralytic ileus.
- Stress response post-burn releases catecholamines and may produce stress (Curling's) ulcers in burns >50 % body surface area.
- Renal complications are predominantly caused by hypovolemia. If perfusion remains poor, high circulating levels of haemoglobin and myoglobin may clog the renal tubules, causing acute tubular necrosis.

8.4.1 Types of Burn Injuries

- *Thermal* (Table 8.4)
  - Dry heat, such as flame and flash
  - Moist heat, such as steam and hot liquids
  - Direct contact, such as hot surfaces and objects

Table 8.4 Causes of thermal burns

Cause	Examples
Dry heat – flame	Clothing catches on fire
	Skin exposed to direct flame
Dry heat – flash	Flame burn associated with explosion (combustible fuels)
Moist heat – hot liquids (scalds)	Bath water
	Beverages – coffee, tea, soup
	Cooking liquids or grease
Moist heat – steam	Pressure cooker
	Microwaved food
	Overheated car radiator
Contact – hot surfaces	Oven burner and door
	Barbecue grill
Contact – hot objects	Tar
	Curling iron
	Cooking pots/pans

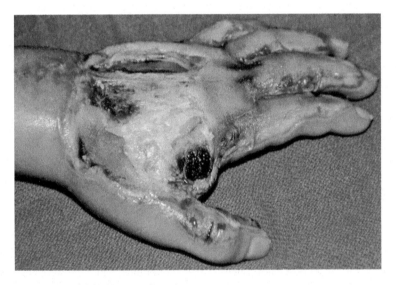

Fig. 8.3 Third degree/full-thickness flame burn

- Major source of morbidity and mortality across all age groups (Figs. 8.3 and 8.4)
- *Chemical* (Fig. 8.5)
  - More than 25,000 chemicals worldwide
  - Divided into two major groups: acids and alkalis
  - Extent and depth injury: directly proportional to the amount, type and strength of the agent, its concentration, degree of penetration, mechanism of action and length of contact time with the skin
- *Electrical* (Fig. 8.6)
  - Comprise a small portion of the burn population.

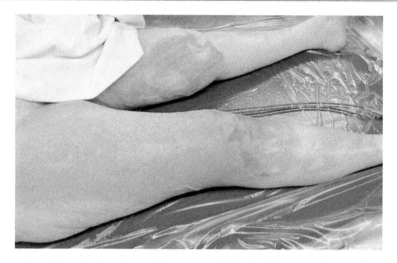

Fig. 8.4 Scald burn: looks can be deceiving – burn wound progression over several days

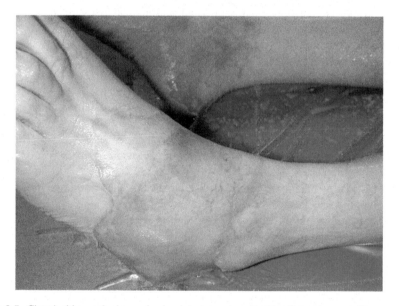

Fig. 8.5 Chemical burns: looks can be deceiving – copious flushing for up to several hours

- Outcomes can be devastating due to tissue damage and potential limb loss.
- Severity of injury difficult to determine as most of the damage may be below skin at level of muscle, fat and bone.
- Entry and exit points determine probable path of current and potential areas of injury.

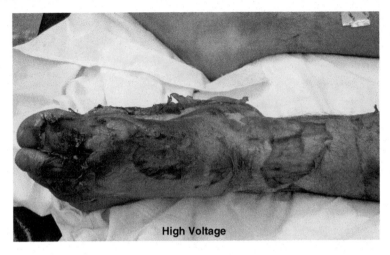

Fig. 8.6 Electrical burn

- If person has fallen post-injury, protect head and cervical spine during transport; need to perform spinal x-rays and neurological assessment.
- May continue to be at risk for cardiac arrhythmias for 24 h post-burn, so ECG needed on admission and at 24 h post-burn.
- Infuse Lactated Ringer's solution at a rate that maintains a good urinary output between 75 and 100 mL/h until colour of urine sufficient to suggest adequate dilution of haemoglobin and myoglobin pigments.
- Administer osmotic diuretic (e.g. mannitol) to establish and maintain acceptable urinary output.
- *Smoke and Inhalation Injury* (Fig. 8.7)
  - Exposure to smoke and inhalation of hot air, steam or noxious products of combustion.
  - Presence of inhalation injury, with a large burn, can double or triple one's mortality rate.
  - Signs and symptoms: burns to head and neck, singed nasal hairs, darkened oral and nasal membranes, carbonaceous sputum, stridor, hoarseness, difficulty swallowing, history of being burned in an enclosed space, exposure to flame, including clothing catching fire near the face, indoors and outdoors.
  - Critical period is 24–48 h post-burn.
  - Most fatalities at fire scene caused by carbon monoxide poisoning or asphyxiation (Table 8.5).
  - Treatment is 100 % humidified oxygen until carboxyhemoglobin falls to acceptable levels.
- *Radiation*
  - Overexposure to sun or radiant heat sources, such as tanning lamps or tanning beds.
  - Nuclear radiation burns require government intervention and specialised treatment.

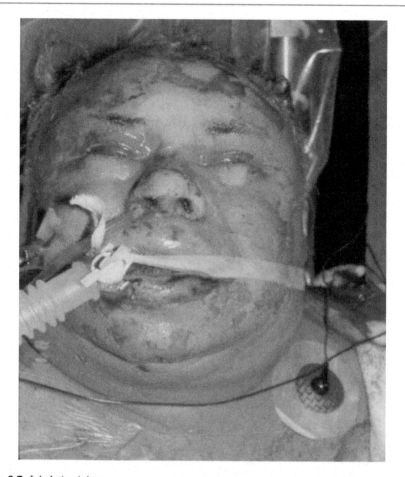

Fig. 8.7 Inhalation injury

Table 8.5 Signs and symptoms of carbon monoxide poisoning

Carboxyhemoglobin saturation (%)	Signs and symptoms
5–10	Visual acuity impairment
11–20	Flushing, headache
21–30	Nausea, impaired dexterity
31–40	Vomiting, dizziness, syncope
41–50	Tachypnea, tachycardia
>50	Coma, death

8.4.1.1 Clinical Manifestations

Care Priorities During the Emergent, Acute and Rehabilitative Periods

1. Principles of care for the *emergent* period: resolution of the immediate problems resulting from the burn injury. The time required for this to occur is usually 1–2 days. The emergent phase ends with the onset of spontaneous diuresis.

2. Principles of care for the *acute* period: avoidance, detection and treatment of complications and wound care. This second phase of care ends when the majority of burn wounds have healed.

3. Principles of care for the *rehabilitative* period: eventual return of the burn survivor to an acceptable place in society and completion of functional and cosmetic reconstruction. This phase ends when there is complete resolution of any outstanding clinical problems resulting from the burn injury.

   • Initial assessment of the burn patient is like that of any trauma patient and can best be remembered by the simple acronym "ABCDEF" (Box 8.2). During the *emergent period*, burn patients exhibit signs and symptoms of hypovolemic shock (Box 8.3). Lack of circulating fluid volumes will also result in minimal urinary output and absence of bowel sounds. The patient may also be shivering due to heat loss, pain and anxiety. With inhalation injury, the airway should be examined visually and then with a laryngoscope/bronchoscope (Box 8.4). The patient may also experience pain, as exhibited by facial grimacing, withdrawing and moaning when touched, particularly if the injuries are partial-thickness in nature. Some areas of full-thickness burn may be anaesthetic to pain and touch if the nerve endings have been destroyed. It is

Box 8.2. Primary Survey Assessment

A	➲	Airway
B	➲	Breathing
C	➲	Circulation
		C-spine immobilisation
		Cardiac status
D	➲	Disability
		Neurological **Deficit**
E	➲	Expose and evaluate
F	➲	Fluid resuscitation

Box 8.3. Signs and Symptoms of Hypovolemic Shock
- Restlessness, anxiety
- Skin – pale, cold, clammy
- Temperature below 37 °C
- Pulse is weak, rapid, ↓ systolic BP
- Urinary output <20 mL/h
- Urine specific gravity >1.025
- Thirst
- Haematocrit <35; BUN ↑

Box 8.4. Physical Findings of Inhalation Injury
- Carbonaceous sputum
- Facial burns, singed nasal hairs
- Agitation, tachypnoea, general signs of hypoxemia
- Signs of respiratory difficulty
- Hoarseness, brassy cough
- Rales, ronchi
- Erythema of oropharynx or nasopharynx

Box 8.5. Signs and Symptoms of Vascular Compromise
- Cyanosis
- Deep tissue pain
- Progressive paraesthesias
- Diminished or absent pulses
- Sensation of cold extremities

Box 8.6. Secondary Survey Assessment
- Head-to-toe examination
- Rule out associated injuries
- Pertinent history
  - Circumstances of injury
  - Medical history

important to examine areas of circumferential full-thickness burn for signs and symptoms of vascular compromise, particularly the extremities (Box 8.5). Areas of partial-thickness burn appear reddened, blistered and oedematous. Full-thickness burns may be dark red, brown, charred black or white in colour. The texture is tough and leathery, and no blisters are present. If the patient is confused, one has to determine if it is the result of hypovolemic shock, inhalation injury, substance abuse, pre-existing history or, more rarely, head injury sustained at the time of the trauma. It is essential to immobilise the c-spines until a full assessment can be performed and the c-spines cleared. At this time, a secondary survey assessment is performed (Box 8.6).
- In the *acute phase*, the focus is on *wound care* and *prevention/management of complications*. At this point, the burn wounds should have declared themselves as being partial-thickness or full-thickness in nature. Eschar on partial-thickness wounds is thinner, and, with dressing changes, it should be possible to see evidence of eschar separating from the viable wound bed.

Healthy, granulation tissue is apparent on the clean wound bed, and re-epithelialising cells are seen to migrate from the wound edges and the dermal bed to slowly close the wound within 10–14 days. Full-thickness wounds have a thicker, more leathery eschar, which does not separate easily from the viable wound bed. Those wounds require surgical excision and grafting. Continuous assessment of the patient's systemic response to the burn injury is an essential part of an individualised plan of care. Subtle changes quickly identified by the burn team can prevent complications from occurring or worsening over time.

- During the final, *rehabilitative phase*, attention turns to *scar maturation, contracture development and functional independence issues*. The areas of burn, which heal either by primary intention or skin grafting, initially appear red or pink and are flat. Layers of re-epithelialising cells continue to form, and collagen fibres in the lower scar tissue add strength to a fragile wound. Over the next month, the scars may become more red from increased blood supply and more raised from disorganised whorls of collagen and fibroblasts/ myofibroblasts. The scars are referred to as hypertrophic in nature. If oppositional forces are not applied through splinting devices, exercises or stretching routines, this new tissue continues to heal by shortening and forming contractures. A certain amount of contracture development is unavoidable, but the impact can be lessened through prompt and aggressive interventions.

8.5   Clinical Management

8.5.1   Nonsurgical Care

Emergent Phase Priorities: airway management, fluid therapy, initial wound care
Emergent Phase Goals of Care: initial assessment, management and stabilisation of the patient during the first 48 h post-burn
Emergent Phase Assessment

- During the rapid, primary survey, airway and breathing assume top priority. A compromised airway requires prompt attention and breath sounds verified in each lung field.
- If circumferential, full-thickness burns are present on the upper trunk and back, ventilation must be closely monitored as breathing might be impaired and releasing escharotomies necessary (Fig. 8.8).
- Spine must be stabilised until c-spines are cleared.
- Circulation is assessed by examining skin colour, sensation, peripheral pulses and capillary filling. Circumferential, full-thickness burns to the arms or legs must be assessed via palpation or Doppler for evidence of adequate circulation. Escharotomies might be required.
- Typically, burn patients are alert and oriented the first few hours post-burn. If that is not the case, consideration must be given to associated head injury

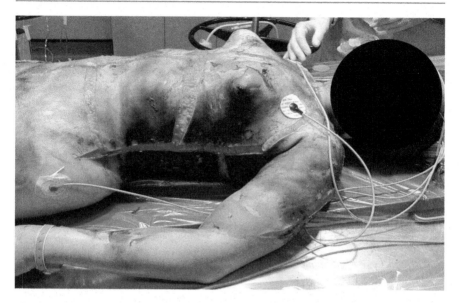

Fig. 8.8 Full-thickness flame burn with releasing escharotomies

(including a complete neurological assessment), substance abuse, hypoxia or pre-existing medical conditions.

- All clothing and jewellery need to be removed in order to visualise the entire body and avoid the "tourniquet-like" effect of constricting items left in place as oedema increases.
- Adherent clothing needs to be gently soaked off with normal saline to avoid further trauma and unnecessary pain.
- Prompt fluid resuscitation must be initiated to address hypovolemic shock.
- Secondary, head-to-toe survey rules out any associated injuries. All medical problems are identified and managed in a timely fashion.
- Circumstances of the injury must be explored to understand the mechanism, duration and severity of the injury.
- Patient's pertinent medical history includes identification of pre-existing disease or associated illness (cardiac or renal disease, diabetes, hypertension), medication/alcohol/drug history, allergies and tetanus immunisation status. A handy mnemonic can be used to remember this information (Box 8.7).

Box 8.7. Secondary Survey Highlights

A	Allergies
M	Medications
P	Previous illness, past medical history
L	Last meal or drink
E	Events preceding injury

Box 8.8. First Aid Management at the Scene

Steps	Action
Step 1	Stop the burning process – remove patient from heat source
Step 2	Maintain airway – resuscitation measures may be necessary
Step 3	Assess for other injuries and check for any bleeding
Step 4	Flush chemical burns copiously with cool water
Step 5	Flush other burns with cool water to comfort
Step 6	Protect wounds from further trauma
Step 7	Provide emotional support and have someone to remain with patient to explain help is on the way
Step 8	Transport the patient as soon as possible to nearby emergency department

Emergent Phase Management

- The top priority of care is to *stop the burning process* (Box 8.8). During the initial first aid period at the scene, the patient must be removed from the heat source, chemicals should be brushed off and/or flushed from the skin, and the patient wrapped in a clean sheet and blanket ready for transport to the nearest hospital. Careful, local cooling of the burn wound with saline-moistened gauze can continue as long as the patient's core temperature is maintained and he/she does not become hypothermic.
  - Upon arrival at the hospital, the burned areas can be cooled further with normal saline, followed by a complete assessment of the patient and initiation of emergency treatment (Box 8.9). In a burn centre, the cooling may take place, using a cart shower system, in a hydrotherapy room (Fig. 8.9). The temperature of the water is adjusted to the patient's comfort level, but tepid is usually best, while the wounds are quickly cleaned and dressings applied.
- *Airway management* includes administration of 100 % oxygen if burns are 20 % body surface area or greater. Suctioning and ventilatory support may be necessary. If the patient is suspected of having or has an inhalation injury, intubation needs to be performed quickly.
- Evidence-based procedures for the insertion of central lines and care of ventilated patients have resulted in impressive reductions in central line blood stream infection rates and ventilator-acquired pneumonia (VAP) [3].
- *Circulatory management* includes intravenous infusion of fluid to counteract the effects of hypovolemic shock for adult patients with burns >15 % body surface area and children with burns >10 % body surface area. Upon admission, two large bore, intravenous catheters should be inserted, preferably into, but not limited to, unburned tissue.

Box 8.9. Treatment of the Severely Burned Patient on Admission

Steps	Action
Step 1	Stop the burning process
Step 2	Establish and maintain an airway; inspect face and neck for singed nasal hair, soot in the mouth or nose, stridor or hoarseness
Step 3	Administer 100 % high-flow humidified oxygen by non-rebreather mask. Be prepared to intubate if respiratory distress increases
Step 4	Establish intravenous line(s) with large bore cannula(e) and initiate fluid replacement using Lactated Ringer's solution
Step 5	Insert an indwelling urinary catheter
Step 6	Insert a nasogastric tube
Step 7	Monitor vital signs including level of consciousness and oxygen saturation
Step 8	Assess and control pain
Step 9	Gently remove clothing and jewellery
Step 10	Examine and treat other associated injuries
Step 11	Assess extremities for pulses, especially with circumferential burns
Step 12	Determine depth and extent of the burn
Step 13	Provide initial wound care – cool the burn and cover with large, dry gauze dressings
Step 14	Prepare to transport to a burn centre as soon as possible

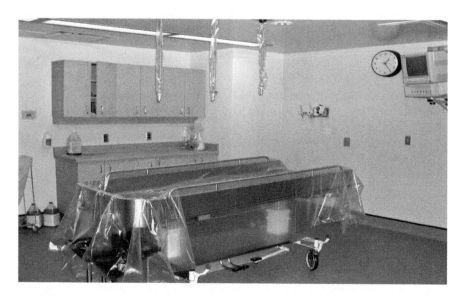

Fig. 8.9 Cart shower for hydrotherapy

- Patients who have large burns where intravenous access will be necessary for a number of days benefit from a central venous access device inserted into either the subclavian, jugular or femoral vein. The overall goal is to establish an access route that will accommodate large volumes of fluid for the first 48 h post-burn.
- The aim of fluid resuscitation is to maintain vital organ function, while avoiding the complications of inadequate or excessive therapy [4]. The most commonly used regimen is the Parkland (Baxter) formula: 4 ml/kg/% body surface area burn using crystalloid (Lactated Ringer's) solution (Box 8.10). *Fluids are calculated for the first 24 h post-burn with "0" hours being the time of the burn,* not *the time of admission to hospital.* One-half of the 24 h total needs to be administered over the first 8 h post-burn, while the remaining half of the estimated resuscitation volume should be administered over the next 16 h.
- It is important to remember that *the formula is only a guideline.* The infusion needs to be adjusted based on the patient's clinical response, which includes vital signs, sensorium and urinary output. For adults, 30–50 mL urine per hour is the goal and 1 mL/kg/h in children weighing less than 30 kg.
- An indwelling urinary catheter needs to be inserted at the same time as the IV's are established in order to reliably measure the adequacy of the fluid resuscitation [5].
- *Wound care.* Wound closure will halt or reverse the various fluid/electrolyte, metabolic and infectious processes associated with an open burn wound. The burns are gently cleansed with normal saline, if the care is being provided on a stretcher or bed. If a hydrotherapy cart shower or immersion tank is used, tepid water cleans the wounds of soot and loose debris (Fig. 8.10). Sterile water is not necessary.

Box 8.10. Fluid Resuscitation Using the Parkland (Baxter) Formula

Formula	Administration	Example
4 mL lactated Ringer's solution per kg body weight per % total body surface area (TBSA) burn = total fluid requirements for the first 24 h post-burn (0 h = time of injury)	½ total in first 8 h	For a 65 kg patient with a 40 % burn injured at 1,000 h:
	¼ total in second 8 h	4 mL × 65 kg × 40 % burn = 10,400 mL in first 24 h
	¼ total in third 8 h	½ total in first 8 h (1,000–1,800 h) = 5,200 mL (650 mL/h)
		¼ total in second 8 h (1,800–0,200 h) = 2,600 mL (325 mL/h)
		¼ total in third 8 h (0,200–1,000 h) = 2,600 mL (325 mL/h)

N.B. Remember that the formula is only a guideline. Titrate to maintain urinary output at 30–50 mL/h, stable vital signs and adequate sensorium

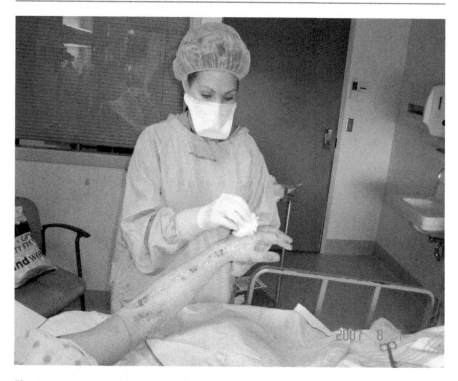

Fig. 8.10 Initial wound care post-admission

- Chemical burns should be flushed copiously for at least 20 min, preferably longer.
- Tar cannot be washed off the wound. It requires numerous applications of an emulsifying agent, such as Tween 80®, Medisol® or Polysporin® ointment.
- During hydrotherapy, loose, necrotic tissue (eschar) may be gently removed (debrided) using sterile scissors and forceps. Hair-bearing areas that are burned should be carefully shaved, with the exception of the eyebrows. Showering or bathing should be limited to 20 min in order to minimise patient heat loss and physical/emotional exhaustion.
- More aggressive debridement should be reserved for the operating room, unless the patient receives conscious sedation.
- After the initial bath or shower, further decisions are made regarding wound care. The frequency of the dressing change depends on the condition of the wound and the properties of the dressing employed. All treatment approaches have certain objectives in common (Table 8.6).

Table 8.6 Objectives of burn wound care

Objective	Rationale
Prevention of conversion	Wounds that dry out or develop an infection can become deeper. A partial-thickness wound could then convert to full-thickness and require skin grafting
Removal of devitalized tissue	Debridement, either through dressing changes or surgery, is necessary to clean the wounds and prepare for spontaneous healing or grafting
Preparation of healthy granulation tissue	Healthy tissue, free of eschar and nourished by a good blood supply, is essential for new skin formation
Minimization of systemic infection	Eschar contains many organisms. Removal is essential in order to decrease the bacterial load and reduce the risk of burn wound infection
Completion of the autografting process	Full-thickness wounds require the application of autologous skin grafts from available donor sites
Limitation of scars and contractures	Wounds that heal well the first time tend to have fewer scars and contractures. Some degree of scar and contracture formation are, however, part of the healing process and cannot be entirely prevented

- Wounds are generally treated with a thin layer of topical antimicrobial cream. Topical coverage is selected according to the condition of the wound, desired results and properties of the topical agent (Table 8.7).
- Assessment criteria have been established for choosing the most appropriate agent (Box 8.11).
- The most commonly selected topical antimicrobial agent is silver sulphadiazene, which can be applied directly to saline-moistened gauze, placed on the wound, covered with additional dry gauze or a burn pad and secured with gauze wrap or flexible netting (Fig. 8.11). These dressings are changed once or twice daily.
- Cartilaginous areas, such as the nose and ears, are usually covered with mafenide acetate (Sulfamylon®), which has greater eschar penetration ability.
- Face care includes the application of warmed, saline-moistened gauze to the face for 20 min, followed by a gentle cleansing and reapplication of a thin layer of ointment, such as polymyxin B sulphate (Polysporin®) (Fig. 8.12).
- Silver-impregnated dressings (Acticoat®/Acticoat® Flex, AQUACEL® Ag) are also commonly used in the emergent phase of burn wound care. These dressings are moistened with sterile water, placed on a burn wound and left intact anywhere from 3 to 4 days to as long as 21 days, depending on the patient's individual clinical status and particular product.
- The ideal dressing should possess particular criteria (Box 8.12). During the first few days post-burn, wounds are examined to determine actual depth. It usually takes a few days for deep, partial-thickness wounds to "declare" themselves. Scald injuries are almost always deeper than they appear on admission and need to be closely monitored.

Table 8.7 Topical antimicrobial agents used on burn wounds

Product	Preparation	Antimicrobial action	Applications
Silver sulphadiazene (SSD®, Silvadene®, Flamazine®)	1 % water-soluble cream	Broad-spectrum antimicrobial activity Poor solubility with limited diffusion into eschar	*Burn wound*: applied using the open or closed dressing method of wound care
Mafenide acetate (Sulfamylon®)	8.5 % water-soluble cream	Bacteriostatic for gram-positive and gram-negative organisms. Highly soluble and diffuses through the eschar	*Deep partial-thickness and full-thickness burns*: applied using either the open (exposure) or closed (occlusive) dressing method
	5 % solution	Same as above	*Graft site*: saturated dressings are applied
Silver nitrate	0.5 % solution	Broad-spectrum antimicrobial activity Hypotonic solution	*Burn wound or graft site*: Saturated, multilayered dressings are applied to the wound or grafted surface
Petroleum and mineral oil-based antimicrobial ointments (e.g. Neosporin®, Bacitracin®, Polysporin®)	Neosporin® (neomycin, bacitracin, polymyxin B), Bacitracin® (bacitracin zinc), Polysporin® (bacitracin, polymyxin B)	Bactericidal for a variety of gram-positive and gram-negative organisms. Ointments have limited ability to penetrate eschar	*Superficial burn wound*: applied to wound in a thin (1 mm) layer and should be reapplied as needed to keep ointment in contact with wound

Box 8.11. Properties of Topical Antimicrobial Agents
- Readily available
- Pharmacologic stability
- Sensitivity to specific organisms
- Non-toxic
- Cost-effective
- Non-painful on application
- Capability of eschar penetration

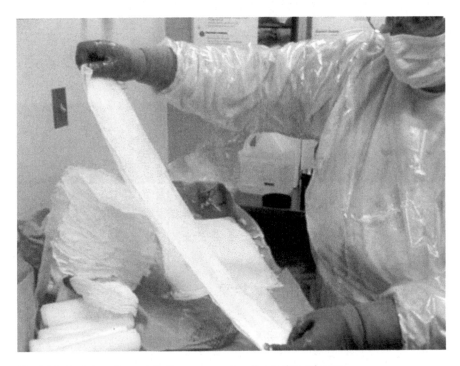

Fig. 8.11 Applying silver sulphadiazene cream to saline-moistened gauze

- Whatever topical and dressing strategies are chosen, basic aseptic wound management techniques must be followed [6]. Personnel need to wear isolation gowns over scrub suits, masks, head covers and clean, disposable gloves to remove soiled dressings or cleanse wounds. Sterile gloves should be used when applying inner dressings or ointment to the face.

Acute Phase Priorities: closure of the burn wound, management of any complications
Acute Phase Goals of Care: spontaneous diuresis, ongoing fluid management, wound closure, detection and treatment of complications over a period of a week to many months, optimal pain management and nutrition

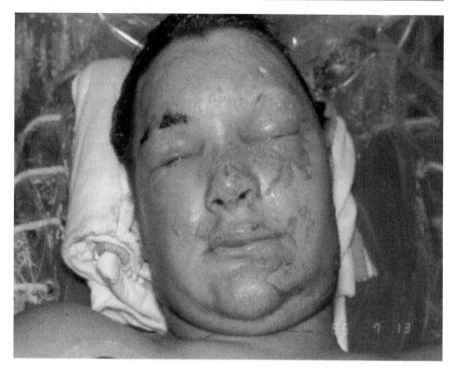

Fig. 8.12 Facial burn wound care

Box 8.12. Criteria for Burn Wound Coverings
- Absence of antigenicity
- Tissue compatibility
- Absence of local and systemic toxicity
- Water vapour transmission similar to normal skin
- Impermeability to exogenous microorganisms
- Rapid and sustained adherence to wound surface
- Inner surface structure that permits ingrowth of fibrovascular tissue
- Flexibility and pliability to permit conformation to irregular wound surface, elasticity to permit motion of underlying body tissue
- Resistance to linear and shear stresses
- Prevention of proliferation of wound surface flora and reduction of bacterial density of the wound
- Tensile strength to resist fragmentation and retention of membrane fragments when removed
- Biodegradability (important for "permanently" implanted membranes)
- Low cost
- Indefinite shelf life
- Minimal storage requirements and easy delivery

Acute Phase Assessment
- Fluid therapy is administered in accordance with the patient's fluid losses and medication administration.
- Wounds are examined on a daily basis, and adjustments are made to the dressings applied. If a wound is full-thickness, arrangements need to be made to take the patient to the operating room for surgical excision and grafting.
- Pain and anxiety levels need to be measured and responded to on a daily basis. A variety of pharmacologic strategies are available (Table 8.8) and address both the background discomfort from burn injury itself and the pain inflicted during procedural and rehabilitative activities.
- Calorie needs are assessed on a daily basis and nutrition adjusted accordingly.

Acute Phase Management
- Wound care is performed daily and treatments adjusted according to the changing condition of the wounds (Table 8.9). Selecting the most appropriate method to close the burn wound is by far the most important task in the acute period. During the dressing changes, nurses debride small amounts of loose tissue for a short period of time, ensuring that the patient receives adequate analgesia and sedation. As the devitalized burn tissue (eschar) is removed from the areas of partial-thickness burn, the type of dressing selected is based on its ability to promote moist wound healing. There are biologic, biosynthetic and synthetic dressings and skin substitutes available today (Table 8.10). Areas of full-thickness damage require surgical excision and skin grafting. There are specific dressings appropriate for grafted areas and donor sites.
- Ongoing rehabilitation, offered through physiotherapy and occupational therapy, is an important part of a patient's daily plan of care. Depending on the patient's particular needs and stage of recovery, there are certain range-of-motion exercises, ambulation activities, chest physiotherapy, stretching and splinting routines to follow. The programme is adjusted on a daily/weekly basis as the patient makes progress towards particular goals and as his/her clinical condition improves or worsens.

Rehabilitative Phase Priorities: maintaining wound closure, scar management, rebuilding strength, transitioning to a rehabilitation facility and/or home

Rehabilitative Phase Goal of Care: returning the burn survivor to a state of optimal physical and psychosocial functioning

Rehabilitation Phase Assessment
- The clinical focus in on ensuring all open wounds eventually close, observing and responding to the development of scars and contractures and ensuring that there is a plan for future reconstructive surgical care if the need exists.

Rehabilitation Phase Management
- Wound care is generally fairly simple at this time. Dressings should be minimal or non-existent. The healed skin is still quite fragile and can break down with very little provocation. The need to moisturise the skin with water-based creams is emphasised in order to keep the skin supple and to decrease the itchiness that may be present.

Table 8.8 Sample burn pain management protocol

Recovery phase	Treatment	Considerations

Critical/acute with mild to moderate pain experience	IV Morphine
	  Continuous infusion, i.e. 2–4 mg q 1 h
	  Bolus for breakthrough, i.e. 1/3 continuous infusion hourly dose
	  Bolus for acutely painful episodes/mobilisation, i.e. 3× continuous infusion hourly dose; consider hydromorphone or fentanyl if morphine ineffective
		Assess patient's level of pain q 1 h using VAS (0–10)
		Assess patient's response to medication and adjust as necessary
		Assess need for antianxiety agents, i.e. Ativan®, Versed®
		Relaxation exercises
		Music distraction

Critical/acute with severe pain experience	1. IV Morphine
	   Continuous infusion for background pain, i.e. 2–4 mg q 1 h
	   Bolus for breakthrough
	2. IV Fentanyl
	   Bolus for painful dressing changes/mobilisation
	3. IV Versed®
	   Bolus for extremely painful dressing change/mobilisation
	4. Propofol Infusion
	   Consult with Department of Anaesthesia for prolonged and extremely painful procedures, i.e. major staple/dressing removal
		Consider fentanyl infusion for short-term management of severe pain
		Assess level of pain q1h using VAS
		Assess level of sedation using SASS score
		Relaxation exercises
		Music distraction
		Assess need for antianxiety/sedation agents, i.e. Ativan®, Versed®

Later acute/rehab with mild to moderate pain experience	Oral continuous release morphine or hydromorphone – for background pain BID Oral morphine or hydromorphone for breakthrough pain and dressing change/mobilisation Consider adjuvant analgesics such as gabapentin, ketoprofen, ibuprofen, acetaminophen	Assess level of pain q1h using VAS Consult equianalgesic table for conversion from IV to PO Assess for pruritus

Table 8.9 Sample burn wound management protocol

Wound status	Treatment	Considerations
Early acute, partial or full thickness, eschar/blisters present	Silver sulphadiazene-impregnated gauze	Apply thin layer (2–3 mm) of silver sulphadiazene to avoid excessive build-up
	Saline-moistened gauze	Monitor for local signs of infection, i.e. purulent drainage and odour, and notify M.D. re. potential need for alternative topical agents, i.e. acetic acid and mafenide acetate
	Dry gauze – outer wrap	
	Mafenide acetate (Sulfamylon®) to cartilaginous areas of face, i.e. nose, ears	
	Polymyxin B sulphate (Polysporin®) to face	
	Change BID to body, face care q4h	
Mid-acute, partial or full thickness, leathery or cheesy eschar remaining	Saline-moistened gauze	Saline dressings to be applied to a relatively small area due to potentially painful nature of treatment
	Dry gauze – outer wrap	Potential use of enzymatic debriding agents (Collagenase Santyl®, Elase®, Accuzyme®)
	Change BID	Monitor for local signs of infection and notify MD
	Full-thickness wounds to be excised surgically	
Late acute, clean partial-thickness wound bed	Non-adherent greasy gauze dressing (Jelonet®, Adaptic®)	Monitor for local signs of infection and notify MD
	Saline-moistened gauze	
	Dry gauze – outer wrap	
	Change once daily	
Post-op graft site	Non-adherent greasy gauze dressing (Jelonet®, Adaptic®)	Select appropriate pressure-relieving sleep surface
	Saline-moistened gauze	Monitor for local signs of infection and notify MD
	Dry gauze – outer wrap	
	Leave intact ×2 days	
	Post-op day 2, gently debulk to non-adherent gauze layer→redress once daily	
	Post-op day 5, gently debulk to grafted area	
	Redress once daily	

Site	Treatment	Notes
Early rehab, healed partial-thickness or graft site	Polymyxin B sulphate (Polysporin®) until wound stable BID When stable, moisturising cream applied BID and prn	Apply thin layer (2 mm) of Polysporin® to avoid excessive build-up Avoid lanolin and mineral-oil containing creams which clog epidermal pores and do not reach dry, dermal layer
Post-op donor site	Hydrophilic foam dressing (i.e. Allevyn®/Mepilex®) or medicated greasy gauze dressing (i.e. Xeroform®) Cover foam with transparent film dressing and pressure wrap ×24 h Remove wrap and leave dressing intact until day 4; replace on day 4 and leave intact until day 8. Remove and inspect If wound unhealed, reapply a second foam dressing If healed, apply polymyxin B sulphate (Polysporin®) BID When stable, apply moisturising cream BID and prn Cover Xeroform® with dry gauze and secure. Leave intact for 5 days Remove outer gauze on day 5 and leave open to air. Apply light layer of polymyxin B sulphate (Polysporin®) ointment. If moist, reapply gauze dressing for 2–3 more days When Xeroform® dressing lifts up as donor site heals, trim excess and apply polymyxin B sulphate (Polysporin®) ointment	Monitor for local signs of infection and notify MD
Face	Normal saline-moistened gauze soaks applied to face ×15 min Remove debris gently using gauze Apply thin layer of polymyxin B sulphate (Polysporin®) Repeat soaks q 4–6 h Apply light layer of mafenide acetate (Sulfamylon®) cream to burned ears and nose cartilage	For male patients, carefully shave beard area on admission and as necessary to avoid build-up of debris. Scalp hair may also need to be clipped carefully on admission to inspect for any burn wounds

Table 8.10 Temporary and permanent skin substitutes

Biological	Biosynthetic	Synthetic
Temporary	Temporary	Temporary
Allograft/homograft (cadaver skin) Clean, partial- and full-thickness burns	Nylon polymer bonded to silicone membrane with collagenous porcine peptides (BioBrane®) Clean, partial-thickness burns, donor sites	Polyurethane and polyethylene thin film (OpSite®, Tegaderm®, Omiderm®, Bioclusive®) Composite polymeric foam (Allevyn®, Mepilex®, Curafoam®, Lyofoam®) Clean, partial-thickness burns, donor sites
Amniotic membrane Clean, partial-thickness burns	Calcium alginate from brown seaweed (Curasorb®, Kalginate®) Exudative wounds, donor sites	Non-adherent gauze (Jelonet®, Xeroform®, Adaptic®) Clean partial-thickness burns, skin grafts, donor sites
Xenograft (pigskin) Clean partial- and full-thickness burns	Human dermal fibroblasts cultured onto BioBrane® (TransCyte®) Clean, partial-thickness burns	
	Mesh matrix of oat beta-glucan and collagen attached to gas-permeable polymer (BGC Matrix®) Clean, partial-thickness burns, donor sites	
Semi-permanent	Semi-permanent	
Mixed allograft seeded onto widely meshed autograft Clean, full-thickness burns	Bilaminar membrane of bovine collagen and glycosaminoglycan attached to Silastic layer (Integra®) Clean, full-thickness burns	
Permanent		
Cultured epithelial autografts (CEA) grown from patient's own keratinocytes (Epicel®) Clean, full-thickness burns		
Allograft dermis decellularized, freeze-dried and covered with thin autograft or cultured keratinocytes (AlloDerm®) Clean, full-thickness burns		

- Visits to outpatient burn clinic provide opportunities for ongoing contact between staff, patients and family post-discharge, wound evaluation and assessment of physical and psychological recovery.
- Scar maturation begins and contractures may worsen. Scar management techniques, including pressure garments, inserts, massage and stretching exercises, need to be taught to patients, and their importance reinforced with each and every visit.
- Encouragement is also essential in order to keep patients and families motivated, particularly during the times when progress is slow and there seems to be no end in sight to the months of therapy.
- The burn surgeon can also plan future reconstructive surgeries for the patient, taking into consideration what improvements the burn patient wishes to see first.

8.5.2 Surgical Care

- Full-thickness burn wounds do not have sufficient numbers of skin-reproducing cells in the dermis to satisfactorily heal on their own. Surgical closure is needed.
- Common practice in surgical burn management is to begin surgically removing (excising) full-thickness burn wounds within a week of admission. Most patients undergo excision of non-viable tissue (Fig. 8.13) and grafting in the same operative procedure. In some instances, if there is concern the wound bed may not be

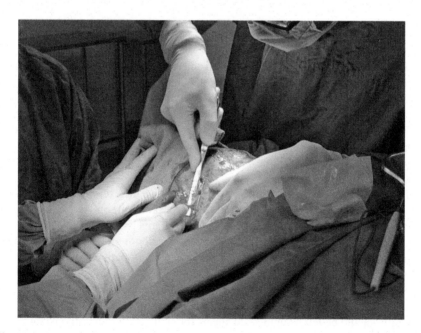

Fig. 8.13 Surgical excision of full-thickness burn wound

Fig. 8.14 Harvesting a
split-thickness skin graft.
Adrenalin/saline soaks may
be applied to donor sites to
control bleeding before the
donor dressing is applied.
Tumescence. Electrocautery
may also be used

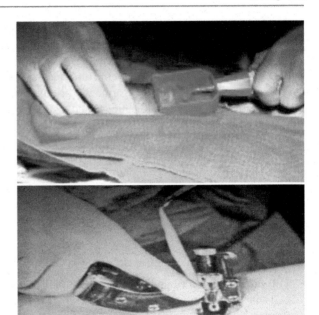

ready for a graft, the wounds are excised and covered with topical antimicrobials, followed by a temporary biologic or synthetic dressing.

- Patient preparation preoperatively includes educational and psychological support to ensure an optimal recovery period postoperatively.
- The donor skin (skin graft), which is harvested in this first O.R., using a dermatome (Fig. 8.14), is then wrapped up in sterile fashion and placed in a skin fridge for later application. Allograft (cadaver skin) may be laid down temporarily.
- Two days later, the patient returns to the OR to have the excised wounds (recipient bed) examined and the donor skin laid as a skin graft on the clean recipient bed. Dressings remain intact for 5 days postoperatively.
- Concern over blood loss and lack of sufficient donor sites are the two limiting factors when attempting to excise and graft patients with extensive wounds.
- Grafts can be split-thickness or full-thickness in depth, meshed or unmeshed in appearance and temporary or permanent in nature (Table 8.11).
- Grafts should be left as unmeshed sheets for application to highly visible areas, such as the face, neck or back of the hand (Fig. 8.15).

Table 8.11 Sources of skin grafts

Type	Source	Coverage
Autograft	Patient's own skin	Permanent
Isograft	Identical twin's skin	Permanent
Allograft/homograft	Cadaver skin	Temporary
Xenograft/heterograft	Pigskin, amnion	Temporary

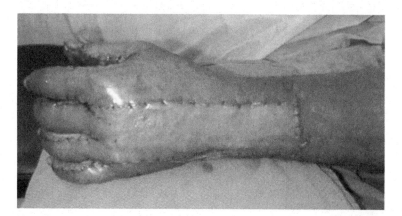

Fig. 8.15 Unmeshed split-thickness sheet graft

- Sheet grafts are generally left open and frequently observed by nursing and medical staff for evidence of serosanguinous exudate under the skin.
- On other parts of the body, grafts can be meshed using a dermatome mesher (Fig. 8.16). The mesher is set to an expansion ratio chosen by the surgeon. An expansion ratio of 1.5:1 allows for exudate to come through and be wicked into a protective dressing, while at the same time be cosmetically acceptable (Fig. 8.17). Wider expansion ratios (3:1, 6:1) allow for increased coverage when there are limited donor sites.
- Meshed skin grafts are generally covered with one of a number of possible options, including silver-impregnated, vacuum-assisted closure, greasy gauze or cotton gauze dressings. Most are left intact for 5 days to allow for good vascularisation between the recipient bed and the skin graft.
- Following the initial "take down" at post-op day 5, the dressings are changed every day until the graft has become adherent and stable, usually around day 8.
- For the next year or so post-burn, the skin grafts mature and their appearance improves (Fig. 8.18). Patients are cautioned that the skin graft appearance will "mature" over the next year and not to be overly concerned about the postoperative appearance.
- The donor site can be dressed with either a transparent occlusive, hydrophilic foam or greasy gauze dressing (Fig. 8.19). Donor sites generally heal in 10–14 days and can be reharvested, if necessary, at subsequent operative procedures (Fig. 8.20). Patients are provided with adequate pain management and support as donor sites are very painful.

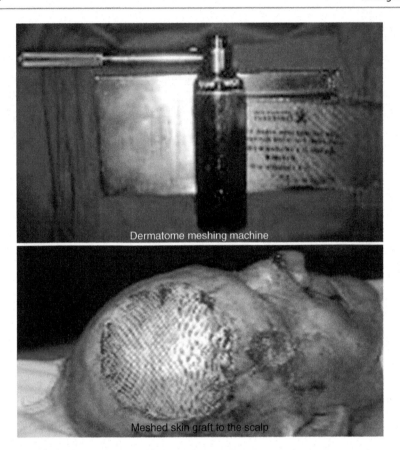

Fig. 8.16 Putting a skin graft through a dermatome mesher. Once harvested, graft is placed on a plastic dermatome carrier and run through a meshing machine. Mesh ratio pattern from 1.5:1 (most common) to 12:1. If donor sites are few and area to cover is large, meshing ratio will increase to 3:1 or 6:1. Exudate can come up through the holes in the mesh pattern to be wicked into the intact dressing. Grafts to the face and hands are not meshed for optimal cosmetic results. These sheet grafts are nursed open

- Over the past 10 years, there have been major advancements in the development, manufacture and clinical application of a number of temporary and permanent biologic skin substitutes. Most of these products were initially developed in response to the problems faced when grafting the massive (i.e. >70 %) burn wound where donor sites are limited (Table 8.12). The search for a permanent skin substitute continues.

8.5.3   Pharmacological Support

Burn patients are assessed for:
- Tetanus toxoid, because of the risk of anaerobic burn wound contamination. Tetanus immunoglobulin is given to those patients who have not been actively immunised within the previous 10 years.

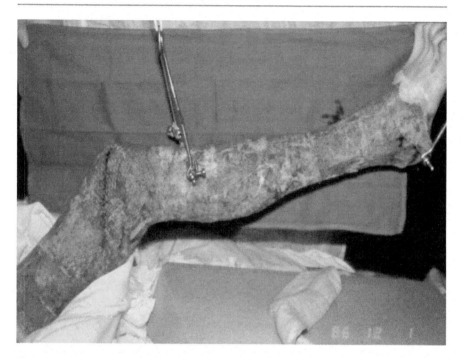

Fig. 8.17 Meshed split-thickness skin graft

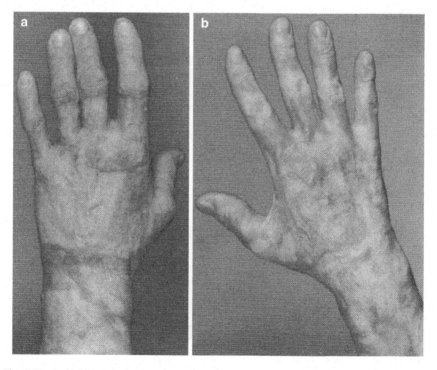

Fig. 8.18 (**a**, **b**) Mature split-thickness skin graft

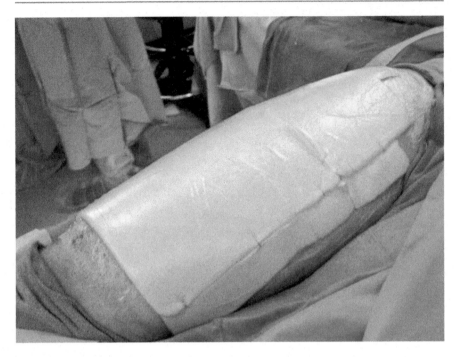

Fig. 8.19 Harvested donor site

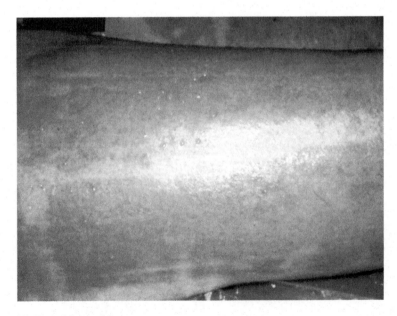

Fig. 8.20 Healed donor site

Table 8.12 Biologic skin replacements

Source	Product	Description
Cultured epithelial autograft (CEA)	Epicel® (Genzyme Corporation, Massachusetts)	Cultured, autologous keratinocytes grown from patient's donated skin cells
		6–8 cells thick, 2–3 weeks culture time
		Lacks dermal component; susceptible to infection
		Lacks epidermal cell-to-connective tissue attachment and is, therefore, very fragile
Dermal replacement	Integra® (Johnson & Johnson, Texas)	Synthetic, dermal substitute
		Neodermis formed by fibrovascular ingrowth of wound bed into 2 mm thick glycosaminoglycan matrix dermal analogue
		Epidermal component, Silastic, removed in 2–3 weeks and replaced with ultrathin autograft
		Functional burn wound cover
		Requires 2 O.R.'s : 1 for dermal placement, 1 for epidermal graft
Dermal replacement	AlloDerm® (LifeCell Corporation, Texas)	Cadaver allograft dermis rendered acellular and nonimmunogenic
		Covered with autograft in same O.R. procedure

Table 8.13 Anxiolytics commonly used in burn care

Generalised anxiety	Situational anxiety (dressing changes, major procedures)	Delirium
Lorazepam (Ativan®) IV	Midazolam (Versed®) IV	Haloperidol (Haldol®) IV
Works nicely in combination with analgesics for routine dressing changes and care	Works nicely in combination with analgesics when very painful and prolonged procedures are performed	Works nicely for patients who appear agitated or disoriented

- Pain medication, which should always be administered intravenously during the hypovolemic shock phase as gastrointestinal function is impaired and intramuscular (IM) medications would not be absorbed adequately.
  - The medication of choice for moderate to severe pain management is an opioid, such as morphine or hydromorphone, as they can be given intravenously and orally and are available in fast-acting and slow-release forms (Table 8.8).
  - As the burn wounds close and the patient's pain level increases, reductions in analgesic therapy should occur by careful taper, rather than abrupt discontinuation, of opioids.
- Sedative agents (Table 8.13).
- Non-pharmacologic approaches to pain management (hypnosis, relaxation, imagery).
- Topical antimicrobial therapy for burn wound care (Table 8.7).

Table 8.14 Medications commonly used in burn care

Types and names	Rationale
Gastrointestinal care	
Ranitidine (Zantac®)	Decreases incidence of stress (Curling's) ulcers
Nystatin (Mycostatin®)	Prevents overgrowth of *Candida albicans* in oral mucosa
Milk of magnesia, lactulose, docusate sodium, sennosides, glycerin or bisacodyl suppository	Prevents/corrects opioid-induced constipation
Nutritional care	
Vitamins A, C, E and multivitamins	Promotes wound healing, immune function,
Minerals: selenium, zinc sulphate, iron (ferrous gluconate and sulphate), folic acid, thiamine	haemoglobin formation and cellular integrity

- The most widely used broad-spectrum antimicrobial agent is silver sulphadiazene. Local application on the burn wound is necessary, as systemic antibiotics would not be able to reach the avascular burn wound.
 - Mafenide acetate is indicated for burned ears and noses as it has a greater ability to penetrate through cartilage.
- Systemic antibiotics when a burn wound infection has been clinically diagnosed or other indicators of sepsis are present, such as pneumonia or uncontrolled fever.
- Additional medications to manage gastrointestinal complications treat antibiotic-induced superinfections and boost the patient's metabolic and nutritional status (Table 8.14).

8.5.4 Psychosocial Support

Psychosocial support to burn survivors and their family members is an essential part of their ongoing care. Concern for family provides them with necessary comfort so they, in turn, can be the patient's single most important social support.

The social worker in a burn centre can provide ongoing counselling and emotional support to patients and family members. Assistance in coping with difficult or stressful matters, such as financial concerns, finding accommodation, questions about hospital insurance coverage or ongoing problems at work or home, is also available. Chaplains offer spiritual support during times of crisis and at various points along the road to recovery. For some, the burn injury is a tremendous test of spiritual faith and brings forward troubling questions for which there are no easy answers, such as "Why did this happen to me and to my family?" Coming to terms with this traumatic event allows the burn survivor to move forward in a positive way. Some burn patients were troubled psychologically pre-burn. They may have formal psychiatric diagnoses and/or histories of drug and/or alcohol abuse. For others, the psychological trauma begins with the burn injury. Referral to a psychiatrist or psychologist for supportive psychotherapy and/or medication can make a positive difference in those situations. It is important, however, before such referrals are made, to discuss the situation with the patient (if he/she is considered mentally competent). This disclosure provides the team with an opportunity to share their interpretation of the patient's behaviours and to listen to how the patient views his/her coping abilities and behaviours. The burn patient and his family need to feel supported and not stigmatised by the recommendation to seek psychological support.

In recent years, the role of patient and family support groups has been examined and encouraged by burn team members. The power of the lived experience is profound. The advice and caring that comes from one who truly knows what it is like to survive a burn injury or the family member of one who has been burned is valuable beyond measure [7–9]. Many burn centres are fortunate to have a burn survivor support group affiliated with them. Based in the USA, but with members from around the world, the Phoenix Society has hundreds of area coordinators and volunteers, through the SOAR (Survivors Offering Assistance in Recovery), who meet with burn survivors in their communities and help; however, they can visit http://www.phoenix-society.org or email info@phoenix-society.org or call 1-800-888-2876 (BURN).

School re-entry programmes and burn camps are also widely available through most paediatric burn centres. Additional information can be obtained from the Phoenix Society or from your provincial/state burn unit/centre.

References

1. Centers for Disease Control and Prevention (2012) Fire deaths and injuries: fact sheet. Available at www.bt.cdc.gov, Accessed on Oct 3, 2012
2. American Burn Association (2011) Burn incidence and treatment in the U.S. Fact Sheet – 2011. Available at www.ameriburn.org, Accessed on Oct 3, 2012
3. Latenser BA (2009) Critical care of the burn patient: the first 48 hours. Crit Care Med 37:2819
4. Saffle JR (2007) The phenomenon of "fluid creep" in acute burn resuscitation. J Burn Care Res 28:382
5. Ahrns KS (2004) Fluid resuscitation in burns. Crit Care Nurs Clin North Am 16:75
6. Helvig EI (2005) Burn wound care. In: Lynn-McHale Wiegand DJ, Carlson KK (eds) AACN procedure manual for critical care, 5th edn. Elsevier, St. Louis
7. Kammerer-Quayle BJ (1993) Helping burn survivors face the future. Progressions 5:11
8. Partridge J (1998) Taking up MacGregor's challenge. J Burn Care Rehabil 19:174
9. Blakeney P et al (2008) Psychosocial care of persons with severe burns. Burns 4:433

Electrical Injury, Chemical Burns, and Cold Injury "Frostbite"

9

Shahriar Shahrokhi

9.1 Electrical Injuries

9.1.1 Introduction

Electrical injuries/burns comprise of a small portion of all burn unit admissions approximately <5 %; however, they have devastating consequences and are a common cause of amputations [1–5].

These injuries are divided into high voltage (>1,000 V) and low voltage (<1,000 V), and their severity is based on:

- Voltage (E)
- Current (amperage – I)
- Current type (AC vs. DC)
- Contact time
  Joule's law defines the amount of tissue damage:
  $Power(J) = Current(I)^2 \times Resistance(R)$. The higher the resistance of tissue to current flow, the greater heat generated which results in greater tissue damage. The various modalities by which electricity can cause injury are summarized in Table 9.1. The tissue damage is caused not only by Joule forces but also by electroporation and protein degradation by electro-conformation [6–9]. The cross-sectional area of the

Table 9.1 The types of electrical injury

Electrical contact	Electrical injury caused by current flow against tissue resistance
Arc	Thermal burn caused by arcing of electrical current passing through the air
Flash	Thermal burn from ignition of clothing or surroundings

S. Shahrokhi, MD, FRCSC
Division of Plastic and Reconstructive Surgery,
Ross Tilley Burn Centre, Sunnybrook Health Sciences Centre,
2075 Bayview Ave, Suite D716, Toronto, ON M4N 3M5, Canada
e-mail: shar.shahrokhi@sunnybrook.ca

M.G. Jeschke et al. (eds.), *Burn Care and Treatment*,
DOI 10.1007/978-3-7091-1133-8_9, © Springer-Verlag Wien 2013

tissue also contributes to the severity of injury with greater damage seen in areas with smaller cross-sectional radius (wrists and ankles) [4, 5]. The current is hence responsible for the tissue damage not the voltage.

9.1.2 Diagnosis and Management

High-voltage injuries should be treated as with all traumas beginning with ABCDE primary survey followed by a thorough secondary survey. Up to 15 % of all electrical injuries are associated with other traumatic injuries; most prevalent are the neurologic (traumatic brain injury – TBI) and orthopedic injuries (fractures) [4, 5, 10]. Many of the organ systems are affected by electrical injury, and these sequelae are summarized in Table 9.2.

High-voltage electrical injuries are a predominant male workforce-related injury with significant sequelae and economic cost. There are practice guidelines for the management of these injuries [16]; however, as these injuries have a low rate of occurrence, they are best managed in specialized centers adept to handling the various complications of these injuries.

In comparison, low-voltage electrical injuries (LVEI) are less common and have more varied etiologies and have less devastating initial sequelae. However, LVEI have more frequent long-term sequelae with delayed presentation and nonspecific symptoms [28, 29]. The common sequelae of LVEI are summarized in Table 9.3. These individuals tend to have a lower rate of return to work due to these neurological and psychological sequelae [29].

Table 9.2 The organ system sequelae of electrical injury and proposed management

System	Sequelae	Management
Neurologic/sensory [4, 5, 11–13, 24–27]	Loss of consciousness	Need to monitor patients and have close follow-up for possible delayed presentation
	Traumatic brain injury	
	Motor and sensory deficits (can be delayed)	
	Tympanic membrane rupture	
	Delayed cataracts	
Cardiovascular [14–19]	Arrhythmias, dysrhythmias	Initial ECG, followed by cardiac monitoring for up to 24–48 h based on presence of:
	Myocardial infarction	ECG abnormalities
	Vascular injury (thrombosis)	Cardiac arrest
		Loss of consciousness
		Role of markers of cardiac damage such as troponin, Ck, Ck-MB unknown
Respiratory Abdominal [4, 5]	Pneumothorax	Treat with chest tube
	Blunt abdominal injury	Treat in accordance to the priority of injury as per ATLS and trauma center guidelines
	Evisceration	
	Ileus, gastroparesis	

System	Sequelae	Management
Renal [4, 5, 22, 23]	Myoglobinuria	Increase fluid resuscitation to maintain a urine output of 1 ml/kg/h
	Acute tubular necrosis	Some controversy regarding alkalinization (with sodium bicarbonate infusion) of urine and forced diuresis (with mannitol)
Musculoskeletal [4, 5, 10, 13, 16, 20, 21]	Muscle necrosis Compartment syndrome Rhabdomyolysis Fracture	Compartment decompression as necessary: Progressive neurologic dysfunction Increased compartment pressure Vascular compromise Clinical deterioration from myonecrosis Excision of all nonviable tissue Might require amputation Manage orthopedic injuries with appropriate consultation

Table 9.3 Common neurological and psychological sequelae of LVEI[a]

Neurologic	Numbness (82 %)
	Paresthesias (63 %)
	Pain (54 %)
	Headache (45 %)
	Weakness (45 %)
Psychologic	Anxiety (54 %)
	PTSD (54 %)
	Poor concentration (54 %)

[a]Adapted from Singerman et al. [28]

9.2 Chemical Burns

Chemical burns represent a small portion of cutaneous burns (reported from 3 to 10 %); however, as with electrical injuries, they have dire consequences [30–33]. There are thousands of different chemicals in everyday use, and this section briefly discusses the general principles in the management of these injuries. In general, the severity of the chemical burn is dependent on the concentration, quantity of the agent, the duration of contact, the depth of penetration, and the mechanism of its action [30, 31]. Table 9.4 summarizes the different classes of chemicals and the mechanism by which they cause tissue damage.

The general principles in the treatment of chemical burns begin as with all trauma with ABCDE of primary trauma survey. The specific measures for chemical burns involve the removal of the inciting agent, treatment of systemic toxicity, specific antidotes if necessary, and local wound care [30]. The general principles for the management of chemical burns are summarized in Table 9.5.

Table 9.4 Classes of chemicals and their mechanisms of tissue injury

Class of chemical	Mechanism of tissue injury
Acid	Coagulation necrosis
Alkali	Liquefaction necrosis – deeper penetration and more severe burns
Organic solutions	Dissolve lipid membranes
Inorganic solutions	Direct binding and salt formation

Table 9.5 Management principles for chemical burns

Removal of chemical agent	Removal of involved clothing
	Thorough and copious irrigation with water except for:
	Phenol – wipe off with 50 % polyethylene glycol sponges [34]
	Dry lime – dust off prior to lavage [35, 36]
	Muriatic acid, sulfuric acid – neutralize with soap or lime water [35, 36]
Systemic toxicity	HF acid – hypocalcemia and ventricular fibrillation [37]
	Formic acid – intravascular hemolysis, renal failure, pancreatitis [38]
	Organic solutions and hydrocarbures – liver failure [30]
	Respiratory injury – can occur with all inhaled agents and must be treated in same manner as inhalation injury [30]
Antidotes	Hydrofluoric acid – inject 10 % calcium gluconate sub-eschar
	White phosphorus – lavage with 1–2 % copper sulfate
Wound care	Wound dressing as for thermal burns
	Early excision of nonviable tissue
	Ophthalmology consult for ocular involvement [39, 40] in addition to copious irrigation

9.3   Cold Injury (Frostbite)

Frostbite is part of the spectrum of localized cold injury, which is associated with the greatest amount of tissue destruction. The mechanisms proposed for tissue injury are:

- Cellular death secondary to cold exposure [41, 42, 45]
- Progressive dermal ischemia [41, 42]

The clinical manifestations of frostbite are as a result of thrombotic events secondary to ischemia/reperfusion injury [41–44] and are classified into four degrees:

- First degree – anesthetic central white plaque with peripheral erythema
- Second degree – blisters surrounded by erythema and edema
- Third degree – hemorrhagic blisters followed by eschar
- Fourth degree – necrosis and tissue loss
- The common risk factors associated with development of frostbite are [41, 42, 49]:
- Mental illness
- Alcohol/drug intoxication
- Extreme of age

> **Box 9.1. General Principles in Treatment of Frostbite[a]**
> 1. Admit patient to specialized unit if possible.
> 2. On admission, rapidly rewarm the affected areas in warm water at 40–42 °C for 15–30 min or until thawing is complete.
> 3. On completion of rewarming, treat the affected parts as follows:
>   (a) Debride white blisters and institute topical treatment with aloe vera every 6 h.
>   (b) Leave hemorrhagic blisters intact and institute topical aloe vera every 6 h.
>   (c) Elevate the affected part(s) with splinting as indicated.
>   (d) Administer anti-tetanus prophylaxis.
>   (e) Antibiotics as indicated.
>   (f) Analgesia: opiates as indicated.
>   (g) Administer ibuprofen 400 mg orally every 12 h.
> 4. Prohibit smoking.
> 5. Treat wounds expectantly, allow for demarcation, and treat surgically as indicated.
>
> [a]Adapted from Murphy et al. [41]

- Diabetic/other neuropathy
- Homelessness

In general, the management of these injuries is similar until full demarcation of the depth and extent of injury, which can take up to 4 weeks [41, 42], and is summarized in Box 9.1.

Much has been studied in the utility of novel therapies for treatment of frostbite (anticoagulation, vasodilators, thrombolytics, sympathectomy, and hyperbaric oxygen); however, there is no conclusive data to prove any of them as gold standard for use in the clinical setting [41, 42, 46, 49]. However, some advocate for the use of thrombolytics and ability to salvage digits [49]. The use of technetium scintigraphy in assessing the extent of tissue damage is becoming widespread and can allow for improved surgical outcome [41, 42, 47–49].

The above-mentioned therapies and medical interventions are key in the treatment of frostbite and can reserve surgical intervention for when absolutely indicated. The main treatment plan is: wait and see.

References

1. Lee RC (1997) Injury by electrical forces: pathophysiology, manifestations and therapy. Curr Probl Surg 34:738–740
2. Esselman PC, Thombs BD, Magyar-Russell G et al (2006) Burn rehabilitation: state of the science. Am J Phys Med Rehabil 85:383–418

3. Purdue GF, Arnoldo BD, Hunt JL (2007) Electric injuries. In: Herndon DN (ed) Total burn care: text and atlas, 3rd edn. Elsevier, Philadelphia, pp 513–520
4. Arnoldo BD, Purdue GF, Kowalske K et al (2004) Electrical injuries: a 20-year review. J Burn Care Rehabil 25:479–484
5. Arnoldo BD, Purdue GF (2009) The diagnosis and management of electrical injuries. Hand Clin 25:469–479
6. Lee RC, Zhang D, Hannig J (2000) Biophysical injury mechanisms in electrical shock trauma. Annu Rev Biomed Eng 2:477–509
7. Block TA, Aarsvold JN, Matthews KL, The 1995 Lindberg Award et al (1995) Nonthermally mediated muscle injury and necrosis in electrical trauma. J Burn Care Rehabil 16:581–588
8. DeBono R (1999) A histological analysis of a high voltage electric current injury to an upper limb. Burns 25:541–547
9. Chen W, Lee RC (1994) Altered ion channel conductance and ionic selectivity induced by large imposed membrane potential pulse. Biophys J 67:603–612
10. Layton TR, McMurty JM, McClain EJ et al (1984) Multiple spine fractures from electric injury. J Burn Care Rehabil 5:373–375
11. Helm PA, Johnson ER, Carlton AM (1977) Peripheral neurologic problems in burn patients. Burns 3:123–125
12. Grube B, Heimbach D, Engrave L, Copass M (1990) Neurologic consequences of electrical burns. J Trauma 10:254–258
13. Rai J, Jeschke MG, Barrow RE, Herndon DN (1999) Electrical injuries: a 30-year review. J Trauma 46:933–936
14. Bailey B, Gaudreault P, Thivierge RL (2000) Experience with guidelines for cardiac monitoring after electrical injury in children. Am J Emerg Med 18:671–675
15. Purdue GF, Hunt JL (1986) Electrocardiographic monitoring after electrical injury: necessity or luxury. J Trauma 26:166–167
16. Arnoldo B, Klein M, Gibran NS (2006) Practice guidelines for the management of electrical injuries. J Burn Care Res 27(4):439–447
17. Housinger TA, Green L, Shahangian S, Saffle JR, Warden GD (1985) A prospective study of myocardial damage in electrical injuries. J Trauma 25:122–124
18. Hammond J, Ward CG (1986) Myocardial damage and electrical injuries: significance of early elevation of CPK-MB isoenzymes. South Med J 79:414–416
19. McBride JW, Labrosse KR, McCoy HG, Ahrenholz DH, Solem LD, Goldenberg IF (1986) Is serum creatine kinase-MB in electrically injured patients predictive of myocardial injury. JAMA 255:764–768
20. Mann R, Gibran N, Engrav L, Heimbach D (1996) Is immediate decompression of high voltage electrical injuries to the upper extremity always necessary? J Trauma 40(4):584–589
21. Dosset AB, Hunt JL, Purdue GF, Schlegal JD (1991) Early orthopedic intervention in burn patients. J Trauma 31:888–893
22. Yowler CJ, Fratianne RB (2000) Current status of burn resuscitation. Clin Plast Surg 27(1):1–10
23. Pham TN, Gibran NS (2007) Thermal and electrical injuries. Surg Clin North Am 87:185–206
24. Johnson EV, Klein LB, Skalka HW (1987) Electrical cataracts: a case report and review of literature. Ophthalmic Surg 18:283–285
25. Boozalis GT, Purdue GF, Hunt JP et al (1991) Ocular changes from electrical burn injuries: a literature review and report of cases. J Burn Care Rehabil 5:458–462
26. Saffle JR, Crandall A, Warden GD (1985) Cataracts: a long-term complication of electrical injury. J Trauma 25:17–21
27. Reddy SC (1999) Electrical cataracts: a case report and review of the literature. Eur J Ophthalmol 9:134–138
28. Singerman J, Gomez M, Fish JS (2008) Long-term sequelae of low-voltage electrical injury. J Burn Care Res 29:773–777

29. Fish JS, Theman K, Gomez M (2012) Diagnosis of long-term sequelae after low-voltage electrical injury. J Burn Care Res 33(2):199–205
30. Paolo R, Monge I, Ruiz M, Barret JP (2010) Chemical burns: pathophysiology and treatment. Burns 36:295–304
31. Hardwicke J, Hunter T, Staruch R, Moiemen N (2012) Chemical burns-an historical comparison and review of literature. Burns 38:383–387
32. Wang CY, Su MJ, Chen HC, Ou SY, Liu KW, Hsiao HT (1992) Going deep into chemical burns. Ann Acad Med Singapore 21:677–681
33. Luterman A, Curreri P (1990) Chemical burn injury. In: Jurkiewcz M, Krizek T, Mathes S (eds) Plastic surgery: principles and practice. CV Mosby, St. Louis, pp 1355–1440
34. Saydjari R, Abston S, Desai MH, Herndon DN (1986) Chemical burns. J Burn Care Rehabil 7:404–408
35. Leonard LG, Scheulen JJ, Munster AM (1982) Chemical burns: effect of prompt first aid. J Trauma 22:420–423
36. Cartotto RC, Peters WJ, Neligan PC, Douglas LG, Beeston J (1996) Chemical burns. Can J Surg 39:205–211
37. Sheridan RL, Ryan CM, Quinby WC Jr, Blair J, Tompkins RG, Burke JF (1995) Emergency management of major hydrofluoric acid exposures. Burns 21:62–63
38. Pruitt BA (1990) Chemical injuries: epidemiology, classification and pathophysiology. Presented at the annual meeting of the American Burns Association, Las Vegas, NV 1990
39. Rozenbaum D, Baruchin AM, Dafna Z (1991) Chemical burns of the eye with special reference to alkali burns. Burns 17:136–140
40. Schrage NF, Rihawi R, Frentz M, Reim M (2004) Acute therapy for eye burns. Klin Monatsbl Augenheilkd 221:253–261
41. Murphy JV, Banwell PE, Roberts AH, McGrouther DA (2000) Frostbite: pathogenesis and treatment. J Trauma 48(1):171–178
42. Petrone P, Kuncir EJ, Asensio JA (2003) Surgical management and strategies in the treatment of hypothermia and cold injury. Emerg Med Clin North Am 21:1165–1178
43. Mazur P (1985) Causes of injury in frozen and thawed cells. Fed Proc 24:14–15
44. Merryman HT (1956) Mechanisms of freezing in living cells and tissues. Science 124:515–518
45. Heggers JP, Robson MC, Manavalen K et al (1987) Experimental and clinical observations on frostbite. Ann Emerg Med 16:1056–1062
46. Skolnick AA (1992) Early data suggest clot-dissolving drugs may help save frostbitten limbs from amputation. JAMA 267:2008–2010
47. Ikawa G, dos Santos PA, Yamaguchi KT, Ibello R (1986) Frostbite and bone scanning: the use of 99m-labelled phosphates in demarcating the line of viability in frostbite victims. Orthopedics 9:1257–1261
48. Salimi Z (1985) Frostbite: assessment of tissue viability by scintigraphy. Postgrad Med 77:133–134
49. Mohr WJ, Jenabzadeh K, Ahrenholz DH (2009) Cold injury. Hand Clin 25:481–496

Long-Term Pathophysiology and Consequences of a Burn Including Scarring, HTS, Keloids and Scar Treatment, Rehabilitation, Exercise

10

Gerd G. Gauglitz

10.1 Introduction

The most common etiologies of burn represent flame and scald burns [1]. Scald burns are most common in victims up to 5 years of age [1]. There is a significant percentage of burns in children that are due to child abuse [2]. A number of risk factors have been linked to burn injury including age, location, demographics, and low economic status [3]. People of increased risk for severe burn injury represent young children and elderly as well as patients of impaired judgment and mobility [1]. The available resources in a given community greatly influence morbidity and mortality since lack of adequate resources significantly affects education, rehabilitation, and survival rates for burn victims. To date, the overall survival rate for burns is 94.6 %, but for at risk populations, survival may be nearly impossible [1]. As demonstrated in a recent milestone study by our group, a burn size of roughly 60 % TBSA represents the crucial threshold for postburn morbidity and mortality in a modern pediatric burn care setting [4].

10.2 Pathophysiology

- Severe burn injury is associated with a profound hypermetabolic, hypercatabolic response which persists for up to 2 years postburn.
- The response is characterized by supraphysiologic metabolic rates, hyperdynamic circulation, constitutive muscle and bone catabolism, growth retardation, insulin resistance, and increased risk for infection.

G.G. Gauglitz, MMS, MD
Department of Dermatology and Allergology,
Ludwig Maximilians University,
Frauenlobstr. 9-11, 80337 Munich, Germany
e-mail: gerd.gauglitz@med.uni-muenchen.de

M.G. Jeschke et al. (eds.), *Burn Care and Treatment*,
DOI 10.1007/978-3-7091-1133-8_10, © Springer-Verlag Wien 2013

- Immediately postburn, there is a decrease in metabolism and tissue perfusion, an "ebb" phase, which is quickly followed by a period of increased metabolic rates and hyperdynamic circulation, a "flow" phase.
- The "flow" phase is characterized by profoundly accelerated glycolysis, lipolysis, proteolysis, insulin resistance, liver dysfunction, and decreases of lean body mass and total body mass [5].
- The primary mediators of this response after severe burn injury are catecholamines, corticosteroids, and inflammatory cytokines which are elevated for up to 12 months postburn [6].
- Net loss of protein leads to loss of lean body mass, and severe muscle wasting leads to decreased strength and failure to fully rehabilitate. This loss of protein is directly related to increases in metabolic rate and may persist up to 9 months after critical burn injury [6]. In young burned children, protein loss leads to significant growth retardation for longer than 1 year post-injury.
- Investigation has shown that the glycolytic-gluconeogenic cycling may experience an increase of 250 % during the postburn hypermetabolic response together with an increase of 450 % in triglyceride-fatty acid cycling. Collectively, these changes lead to greater glycogenolysis, gluconeogenesis, and increased circulation of glucogenic precursors, which translates into hyperglycemia and impaired responsiveness to insulin, which is in term related to post-receptor insulin resistance.
- Both serum glucose and insulin increase postburn and remain significantly increased throughout the entire acute hospital stay. These increased amounts of available glucose although required as a source of energy to decrease severe protein catabolism after severe burn injury, if left untreated, have led to poor outcomes in studies performed in critically ill patients [7].
- It was originally thought that these metabolic alterations resolve shortly after burn-wound closure or the acute hospitalization. However, current work demonstrated a long-lasting state of this hypermetabolic response persisting for up to 3 years after burn trauma [8–13].

10.3 Scarring

- Incidence rates of hypertrophic scarring vary from 40 to 70 % following surgery to up to 91 % following burn injury, depending on the depth of the wound [14, 15].
- Excessive scars represent aberrations in the fundamental processes of wound healing, where there is an obvious imbalance between the anabolic and catabolic phases [16].
- Evidence to date strongly implies a prolonged inflammatory period, the consequence of which may contribute to increased fibroblast activity with greater and more sustained ECM deposition [16].
- Burn scars after deep dermal injury are cosmetically disfiguring and force the scarred person to deal with an alteration in body appearance [17]. Multiple studies on excessive scar formation have been conducted for decades and

have led to a plethora of therapeutic strategies in order to prevent or attenuate excessive scar formation postburn [18].

10.4 Therapy

Pressure therapy has been the preferred conservative management for both the prophylaxis and treatment of hypertrophic scars and keloids since the 1970s and is still frequently used for the prophylaxis of hypertrophic burn scar formation [18]:

- Decreased collagen synthesis by limiting the supply of blood, oxygen, and nutrients to the scar tissue [19–21] and increased apoptosis [22] are being discussed as underlying mechanism of action.
- Continuous pressure of 15–40 mmHg for at least 23 h/day for more than 6 months while the scar is still active is currently recommended [20, 23].
- Compression therapy is limited by the ability to adequately fit the garment to the wounded area, and patient discomfort frequently reduces compliance.

Silicone gel sheeting has been a well-established management of scars since its introduction in the early 1980s, and its therapeutic effects on predominantly hypertrophic scars have been well documented in the literature [24, 25]:

- Normalization of occlusion and transepidermal water loss (TEWL) are likely the mechanisms of the therapeutic action of silicone gel sheeting rather than an inherent anti-scarring property of silicone [26].
- Silicone sheets are recommended to be worn for 12 or more hours a day for at least 2 months beginning 2 weeks after wound healing.
- Silicone gel is favored for areas of consistent movement where sheeting will not conform and should be applied twice daily [27].

Intralesional steroid injections have gained popularity as one of the most common approaches to attenuate hypertrophic scar and keloid formation since the mid-1960s [28]:

- Effects of corticosteroids result primarily from its suppressive effects on the inflammatory process in the wound [26] and secondarily, from reduced collagen and glycosaminoglycan synthesis, inhibition of fibroblast growth [29], and enhanced collagen and fibroblast degeneration [30].
- Three to four injections of triamcinolone acetonide (TAC, 10–40 mg/ml) are generally sufficient, although occasionally injections continue for 6 months or more [28].
- Response rates are highly variable, with figures ranging from 50 to 100 % and a recurrence rate of 9–50 % [31].
- When used alone, intralesional corticosteroid injections have the most effect on younger keloids and can provide symptomatic relief.
- For older hypertrophic scars and keloids, combination with cryotherapy (contact or spray cryotherapy with liquid nitrogen) may show more effective results [32, 33] and represents the most widely used modality in our daily practice. Indeed, combination of cryotherapy with intralesional TAC injections seems to yield marked improvement of hypertrophic scars and keloids [34–36].

- We recommend cryotherapy directly before the administration of intralesional TAC injections since success rates appear to be increased based on the larger amount of TAC that can be injected due to edema formation caused by cryotherapy.

Superficial x-rays, electron beam, and low- or high-dose-rate brachytherapy have been used in scar reduction protocols primarily as an adjunct to surgical removal of keloids with good results [37]:

- Radiation is thought to mediate its effects on keloids through inhibition of neo-vascular buds and proliferating fibroblasts, resulting in a decreased amount of collagen produced [26].
- Electron beam irradiation is usually started 24–48 h after keloid excision, and the total dose is limited to 40 Gy over several administrations in order to prevent side effects such as hypo- and hyperpigmentation, erythema, telangiectasia, and atrophy [38].
- Since radiation represents a potential risk in terms of carcinogenesis, particularly in areas such as the breast or thyroid, its use should be handled with caution [39, 40].

In 1999, Fitzpatrick [41] was the first to report on using *5-fluorouracil (5-FU)* to effectively reduce scar in his 9-year experience, administering more than 5,000 injections to more than 1,000 patients. Ever since, the use of intralesional 5-FU in combination or as a sole agent for treatment of keloids has been shown to be effective:

- 5-FU is normally injected weekly at concentrations of 50 mg/ml, continuing for up to 16 weeks.
- Therapy in pregnant women or patients with bone marrow suppression should be avoided.
- Novel approaches include the combination of intralesional application of TAC and 5-FU (mostly mixtures of 75 % 5-FU and 25 % TAC (40 mg/ml) in weekly intervals for 8 weeks) demonstrating superior results to intralesional steroid therapy alone [42–44].

Surgical approaches include various biological and synthetic substrates to replace the injured skin:

- Integra® was found to improve aesthetic outcome postburn in the management of severe full-thickness burns of ≥50 % TBSA in a pediatric patient population compared to standard autograft-allograft technique [45]. It was also found to inhibit scar formation and wound contraction [46].
- Several strategies have been investigated with the purpose of promoting wound healing by the use of gene transfer, including stimulation of the granulation process, the vascularization, the reepithelialization, or the scar quality [47, 48]. However, more studies are needed to define growth factor levels in different phases of wound healing and to elucidate the precise timing of gene expression or downregulation required to better augment wound healing and control of scar formation [49].

10.5 Psychological Aspects

With improvements in mortality, outcomes are increasingly focused on measures of function and community integration [50]. Authors are now reporting new methods to evaluate outcomes through Burn-Specific Health Scales [51] and measures of adjustment:

- Authors found that severely burned adult patients adjust relatively well, although some develop clinically significant psychological disturbances such as somatization and phobic anxiety [52]. Depression and post-traumatic stress disorder (PTSD), which are prevalent in 13–23 % and 13–45 % of cases, respectively, have been the most common areas of research in burn patients [17].

- Risk factors related to depression represent pre-burn depression and female gender in combination with facial disfigurement [17].
- Social problems include difficulties in sexual life and social interactions. The quality of life initially seems to be lower in severely burn patients when compared with the general population [17].
- Children with severe burns were found to have similar somatization problems as well as sleep disturbances but in general, were well adjusted [52].
- These data intimate that major burns can lead to significant disturbances in psychiatric health and outcomes, but in general, these can be overcome.

10.6   Return to Work

The ultimate goal of rehabilitation after burn injury is reintegration into society, which includes employment [53]. A study in 363 burned adults who were employed at the time of injury demonstrated a mean time off work of 17 weeks. Only 37 % returned to the same job, with the same employer, without accommodations in a detailed subgroup analysis [54]. Based on current data, predictors of return to work include the following characteristics:

- TBSA and burn site
- Medical factors such as length of hospitalization and psychiatric history
- Demographic factors including age, race, marital status, and employment status at the time of injury [55–58]

10.7   Long-Term Development of Other Diseases

Burn injury is associated with long-term consequences despite adequate and rapid therapy immediately postburn. Recent data delineated the complexity of the pathophysiologic response postburn and identified derangements that are greater and more protracted than previously thought [6]:

- These data indicate the local and systemic effects of a burn are not limited to the 95 % healed stage [52]. Burn injury continues to plague and impair patients over a prolonged time.
- Given the great adverse events associated with the hypermetabolic and hyperinflammatory responses, prolonged treatment needs for severely burned patients are currently identified.
- Several studies aim to determine whether long-term effects can be alleviated [11, 59–62]. Administration of anabolic agents such as oxandrolone, growth hormone, or propranolol may improve long-term outcomes. Also, exercise can tremendously improve strength and rehabilitation of severely burned patients [63].

10.8 Exercise

A balanced physical therapy program is essential to restore metabolic variables and prevent burn-wound contracture.

Progressive resistance exercises in convalescent burn patients can maintain and improve body mass, augment incorporation of amino acids into muscle proteins, and increase muscle strength and the ability to walk distances by approximately 50 % [64].

10.9 Summary

A burn is not limited to its acute phase. It is a process that continues over a long time and requires a continuing patient-specific treatment plan in order to improve patient outcome.

References

1. Pham TN, Kramer CB, Wang J, Rivara FP, Heimbach DM, Gibran NS, Klein MB (2009) Epidemiology and outcomes of older adults with burn injury: an analysis of the national burn repository. J Burn Care Res 30(1):30–36
2. Andronicus M, Oates RK, Peat J, Spalding S, Martin H (1998) Non-accidental burns in children. Burns 24(6):552–558
3. Fire deaths and injuries: fact sheet. http://www.cdc.gov/HomeandRecreationalSafety/Fire-Prevention/fires-factsheet.html
4. Kraft R, Herndon DN, Al-Mousawi AM, Williams FN, Finnerty CC, Jeschke MG (2012) Burn size and survival probability in paediatric patients in modern burn care: a prospective observational cohort study. Lancet 379(9820):1013–1021
5. Herndon DN, Hart DW, Wolf SE, Chinkes DL, Wolfe RR (2001) Reversal of catabolism by beta-blockade after severe burns. N Engl J Med 345(17):1223–1229
6. Jeschke MG, Chinkes DL, Finnerty CC, Kulp G, Suman OE, Norbury WB, Branski LK, Gauglitz GG, Mlcak RP, Herndon DN (2008) Pathophysiologic response to severe burn injury. Ann Surg 248(3):387–401
7. van den Berghe G, Wouters P, Weekers F, Verwaest C, Bruyninckx F, Schetz M, Vlasselaers D, Ferdinande P, Lauwers P, Bouillon R (2001) Intensive insulin therapy in critically ill patients. N Engl J Med 345(19):1359–1367
8. Jeschke MG, Mlcak RP, Finnerty CC, Norbury WB, Gauglitz GG, Kulp GA, Herndon DN (2007) Burn size determines the inflammatory and hypermetabolic response. Crit Care 11(4):R90
9. Norbury WB, Herndon DN (2007) Modulation of the hypermetabolic response after burn injury. In: Herndon DN (ed) Total burn care, 3rd edn. Saunders/Elsevier, New York, pp 420–433
10. Mlcak RP, Jeschke MG, Barrow RE, Herndon DN (2006) The influence of age and gender on resting energy expenditure in severely burned children. Ann Surg 244(1):121–130
11. Hart DW, Wolf SE, Mlcak R, Chinkes DL, Ramzy PI, Obeng MK, Ferrando AA, Wolfe RR, Herndon DN (2000) Persistence of muscle catabolism after severe burn. Surgery 128(2):312–319
12. Jeschke MG, Gauglitz GG, Kulp GA, Finnerty CC, Williams FN, Kraft R, Suman OE, Mlcak RP, Herndon DN (2011) Long-term persistence of the pathophysiologic response to severe burn injury. PLoS One 6(7):e21245

13. Gauglitz GG, Herndon DN, Kulp GA, Meyer WJ 3rd, Jeschke MG (2009) Abnormal insulin sensitivity persists up to three years in pediatric patients post-burn. J Clin Endocrinol Metabol 94(5):1656–1664

14. Deitch EA, Wheelahan TM, Rose MP, Clothier J, Cotter J (1983) Hypertrophic burn scars: analysis of variables. J Trauma 23(10):895–898

15. Lewis WH, Sun KK (1990) Hypertrophic scar: a genetic hypothesis. Burns 16(3): 176–178

16. Brown JJ, Bayat A (2009) Genetic susceptibility to raised dermal scarring. Br J Dermatol 161(1):8–18

17. Van Loey NE, Van Son MJ (2003) Psychopathology and psychological problems in patients with burn scars: epidemiology and management. Am J Clin Dermatol 4(4): 245–272

18. Gauglitz GG, Korting HC, Pavicic T, Ruzicka T, Jeschke MG (2011) Hypertrophic scarring and keloids: pathomechanisms and current and emerging treatment strategies. Mol Med 17(1–2):113–125

19. Baur PS, Larson DL, Stacey TR, Barratt GF, Dobrkovsky M (1976) Ultrastructural analysis of pressure-treated human hypertrophic scars. J Trauma 16(12):958–967

20. Macintyre L, Baird M (2006) Pressure garments for use in the treatment of hypertrophic scars–a review of the problems associated with their use. Burns 32(1):10–15

21. Kelly AP (2004) Medical and surgical therapies for keloids. Dermatol Ther 17(2):212–218

22. Reno F, Sabbatini M, Lombardi F, Stella M, Pezzuto C, Magliacani G, Cannas M (2003) In vitro mechanical compression induces apoptosis and regulates cytokines release in hypertrophic scars. Wound Repair Regen 11(5):331–336

23. Van den Kerckhove E, Stappaerts K, Fieuws S, Laperre J, Massage P, Flour M, Boeckx W (2005) The assessment of erythema and thickness on burn related scars during pressure garment therapy as a preventive measure for hypertrophic scarring. Burns 31(6):696–702

24. Sawada Y, Sone K (1992) Hydration and occlusion treatment for hypertrophic scars and keloids. Br J Plast Surg 45(8):599–603

25. Fulton JE Jr (1995) Silicone gel sheeting for the prevention and management of evolving hypertrophic and keloid scars. Dermatol Surg 21(11):947–951

26. Reish RG, Eriksson E (2008) Scar treatments: preclinical and clinical studies. J Am Coll Surg 206(4):719–730

27. Slemp AE, Kirschner RE (2006) Keloids and scars: a review of keloids and scars, their pathogenesis, risk factors, and management. Curr Opin Pediatr 18(4):396–402

28. Jalali M, Bayat A (2007) Current use of steroids in management of abnormal raised skin scars. Surgeon 5(3):175–180

29. Cruz NI, Korchin L (1994) Inhibition of human keloid fibroblast growth by isotretinoin and triamcinolone acetonide in vitro. Ann Plast Surg 33(4):401–405

30. Boyadjiev C, Popchristova E, Mazgalova J (1995) Histomorphologic changes in keloids treated with Kenacort. J Trauma 38(2):299–302

31. Robles DT, Berg D (2007) Abnormal wound healing: keloids. Clin Dermatol 25(1):26–32

32. Murray JC (1994) Keloids and hypertrophic scars. Clin Dermatol 12(1):27–37

33. Lawrence WT (1991) In search of the optimal treatment of keloids: report of a series and a review of the literature. Ann Plast Surg 27(2):164–178

34. Boutli-Kasapidou F, Tsakiri A, Anagnostou E, Mourellou O (2005) Hypertrophic and keloidal scars: an approach to polytherapy. Int J Dermatol 44(4):324–327

35. Jaros E, Priborsky J, Klein L (1999) Treatment of keloids and hypertrophic scars with cryotherapy. Acta Medica (Hradec Kralove) Suppl 42(2):61–63

36. Yosipovitch G, Widijanti Sugeng M, Goon A, Chan YH, Goh CL (2001) A comparison of the combined effect of cryotherapy and corticosteroid injections versus corticosteroids and cryotherapy alone on keloids: a controlled study. J Dermatolog Treat 12(2):87–90

37. Guix B, Henriquez I, Andres A, Finestres F, Tello JI, Martinez A (2001) Treatment of keloids by high-dose-rate brachytherapy: a seven-year study. Int J Radiat Oncol Biol Phys 50(1):167–172

38. Ogawa R, Mitsuhashi K, Hyakusoku H, Miyashita T (2003) Postoperative electron-beam irradiation therapy for keloids and hypertrophic scars: retrospective study of 147 cases followed for more than 18 months. Plast Reconstr Surg 111(2):547–555

39. Atiyeh BS (2007) Nonsurgical management of hypertrophic scars: evidence-based therapies, standard practices, and emerging methods. Aesthetic Plast Surg 31(5):468–494

40. Leventhal D, Furr M, Reiter D (2006) Treatment of keloids and hypertrophic scars: a meta-analysis and review of the literature. Arch Facial Plast Surg 8(6):362–368

41. Fitzpatrick RE (1999) Treatment of inflamed hypertrophic scars using intralesional 5-FU. Dermatol Surg 25(3):224–232

42. Davison SP, Dayan JH, Clemens MW, Sonni S, Wang A, Crane A (2009) Efficacy of intralesional 5-fluorouracil and triamcinolone in the treatment of keloids. Aesthet Surg 29(1):40–46

43. Sadeghinia A, Sadeghinia S (2012) Comparison of the efficacy of intralesional triamcinolone acetonide and 5-fluorouracil tattooing for the treatment of keloids. Dermatol Surg 38(1): 104–109

44. Darougheh A, Asilian A, Shariati F (2009) Intralesional triamcinolone alone or in combination with 5-fluorouracil for the treatment of keloid and hypertrophic scars. Clin Exp Dermatol 34(2):219–223

45. Branski LK, Herndon DN, Pereira C, Mlcak RP, Celis MM, Lee JO, Sanford AP, Norbury WB, Zhang XJ, Jeschke MG (2007) Longitudinal assessment of Integra in primary burn management: a randomized pediatric clinical trial. Crit Care Med 35(11):2615–2623

46. Clayman MA, Clayman SM, Mozingo DW (2006) The use of collagen-glycosaminoglycan copolymer (Integra) for the repair of hypertrophic scars and keloids. J Burn Care Res 27(3): 404–409

47. Petrie NC, Vranckx JJ, Hoeller D, Yao F, Eriksson E (2005) Gene delivery of PDGF for wound healing therapy. J Tissue Viability 15(4):16–21

48. Rogers B, Lineaweaver WC (2002) Skin wound healing and cell-mediated DNA transport. J Long Term Eff Med Implants 12(2):125–130

49. Gauglitz GG, Jeschke MG (2011) Combined gene and stem cell therapy for cutaneous wound healing. Mol Pharm 8(5):1471–1479

50. Engrav LH, Covey MH, Dutcher KD, Heimbach DM, Walkinshaw MD, Marvin JA (1987) Impairment, time out of school, and time off from work after burns. Plast Reconstr Surg 79(6):927–934

51. Kildal M, Andersson G, Fugl-Meyer AR, Lannerstam K, Gerdin B (2001) Development of a brief version of the Burn Specific Health Scale (BSHS-B). J Trauma 51(4):740–746

52. Jeschke MG, Williams FN, Gauglitz GG, Herndon DN (2012) Burns. In: Townsend M, Beauchamp RD, Evers MB, Kenneth ML (eds) Sabiston textbook of surgery, vol 19. Elsevier, Philadelphia, p 521

53. Schneider JC, Bassi S, Ryan CM (2011) Employment outcomes after burn injury: a comparison of those burned at work and those burned outside of work. J Burn Care Res 32(2): 294–301

54. Brych SB, Engrav LH, Rivara FP, Ptacek JT, Lezotte DC, Esselman PC, Kowalske KJ, Gibran NS (2001) Time off work and return to work rates after burns: systematic review of the literature and a large two-center series. J Burn Care Rehabil 22(6):401–405

55. Bowden ML, Thomson PD, Prasad JK (1989) Factors influencing return to employment after a burn injury. Arch Phys Med Rehabil 70(10):772–774

56. Dyster-Aas J, Kildal M, Willebrand M (2007) Return to work and health-related quality of life after burn injury. J Rehabil Med 39(1):49–55

57. Moi AL, Wentzel-Larsen T, Salemark L, Hanestad BR (2007) Long-term risk factors for impaired burn-specific health and unemployment in patients with thermal injury. Burns 33(1):37–45

58. Schneider JC, Bassi S, Ryan CM (2009) Barriers impacting employment after burn injury. J Burn Care Res 30(2):294–300

59. Hart DW, Wolf SE, Chinkes DL, Beauford RB, Mlcak RP, Heggers JP, Wolfe RR, Herndon DN (2003) Effects of early excision and aggressive enteral feeding on hypermetabolism, catabolism, and sepsis after severe burn. J Trauma 54(4):755–761; discussion 761–764
60. Hart DW, Wolf SE, Ramzy PI, Chinkes DL, Beauford RB, Ferrando AA, Wolfe RR, Herndon DN (2001) Anabolic effects of oxandrolone after severe burn. Ann Surg 233(4):556–564
61. Herndon DN, Tompkins RG (2004) Support of the metabolic response to burn injury. Lancet 363(9424):1895–1902
62. Przkora R, Herndon DN, Suman OE, Jeschke MG, Meyer WJ, Chinkes DL, Mlcak RP, Huang T, Barrow RE (2006) Beneficial effects of extended growth hormone treatment after hospital discharge in pediatric burn patients. Ann Surg 243(6):796–801; discussion 801–803
63. Al-Mousawi AM, Williams FN, Mlcak RP, Jeschke MG, Herndon DN, Suman OE (2010) Effects of exercise training on resting energy expenditure and lean mass during pediatric burn rehabilitation. J Burn Care Res 31(3):400–408
64. Cucuzzo NA, Ferrando A, Herndon DN (2001) The effects of exercise programming vs traditional outpatient therapy in the rehabilitation of severely burned children. J Burn Care Rehabil 22(3):214–220

Burn Reconstruction Techniques

11

Lars-Peter Kamolz and Stephan Spendel

Due to extraordinary advances concerning the understanding of cellular and molecular processes in wound healing, wound care innovations and new developments concerning burn care have been made; burn care has improved to the extent that persons with burns frequently can survive. The trend in current treatment extends beyond the preservation of life; the ultimate goal is the return of burn victims, as full participants, back into their social and business life [1, 2].

A more aggressive approach in the acute phase has led to a higher survival rates on one side but also to a higher number of patients, who will require reconstructive surgery on the other side. Successful reconstruction requires a profound understanding of skin anatomy and physiology, careful analysis of the defect, and thoughtful considerations of different techniques suitable to execute the surgical plan [3].

11.1 From the Reconstructive Ladder to the Reconstructive Elevator

Based on the concept of the reconstructive ladder by Mathes und Nahai, new advances in the understanding of the anatomy, operative techniques, instrumentation, and surgical skills have led to the concept of the reconstructive elevator: complex procedures are no longer considered as last resort procedures only. In the quest to provide optimal form and function, it is currently accepted to jump several rungs of the ladder due to the knowledge that some defects require more complex solutions. The goal of surgical reconstruction is restoration of preoperative function and appearance. The surgeon must reconstruct the defect with

L.-P. Kamolz, MD, PhD, MSc (✉) • S. Spendel, MD, PhD
Division of Plastic, Aesthetic and Reconstructive Surgery,
Department of Surgery, Medical University of Graz,
Auenbruggerplatz 29, 8036 Graz, Austria
e-mail: lars.kamolz@medunigraz.at

M.G. Jeschke et al. (eds.), *Burn Care and Treatment*,
DOI 10.1007/978-3-7091-1133-8_11, © Springer-Verlag Wien 2013

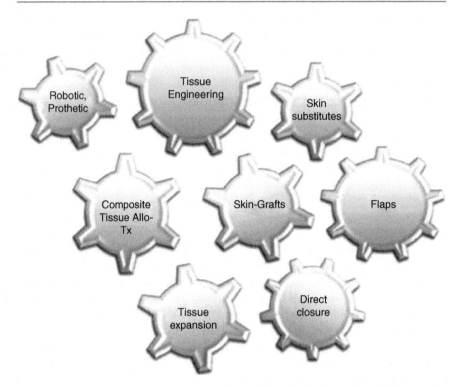

Fig. 11.1 The reconstructive clockwork: the interlocking wheels of a clockwork illustrate the integration of different reconstructive methods

tissues that is missing and which allows defect coverage with tissue of similar contour, texture, and color [4, 5].

11.2 The Reconstructive Clockwork

In clinical daily routine, combinations of different techniques are often applied in order to permit new reconstructive possibilities for the patient, but neither the reconstructive ladders of Mathes and Nahai in 1982 nor the reconstructive elevator permits a real combination of the different reconstructive procedures and techniques.

The image of interlocking wheels of a clockwork [6] (Fig. 11.1) illustrates the integration of different reconstructive methods even more impressive than the conventional reconstructive ladder and elevator.

11.2.1 General Principles

Hypertrophic scars and scar contraction with concomitant functional impairment are the most common problems that require correction or reconstruction. Choosing the right modality depends upon several factors, for example, the age or maturity of the scar. The knowledge of the healing properties of the patient (i.e., whether the patient has a propensity toward keloid or hypertrophic scar production) might also help to dictate how aggressive or how conservative one may wish to pursue the treatment.

Objective assessment of deformities and functional impairment is of utmost importance for planning the right reconstructive procedure. Formulating a realistic plan to restore the functional problems requires analysis of the physical deformities and psychological disturbance of the patient. Psychiatric, psychosocial [7], and physiotherapeutic cares have to be continued while a surgical treatment plan is instituted.

11.3   Indication and Timing of Surgical Intervention

For a surgeon, making a decision *how* to operate on a patient with burn deformities is quite simple. In contrast, deciding *when* to operate on a patient can be difficult. However, the basic principle is based on the following rule:
- Restoring bodily deformities that impose functional difficulties must precede any surgical effort to restore the appearance.

In short, a surgeon's effort must be concentrated upon restoring the deformed bodily parts essential for physical functions, if not for patient survival. In contrast, restoration of deformed regions, in general, can be performed in a later phase.

It is postulated that attempts to correct burn deformities should be delayed for at least 1–2 years. During this time needed for scar maturation, an interim conservative treatment by using pressure garments and splinting is recommended to reduce scarring and to minimize joint contracture because operating on an immature scar is technically more cumbersome and will lead to a higher number of complications. It is never too late to revise a scar, but conversely, it may be too early.

11.4   The Techniques of Reconstruction

There are several techniques routinely used to reconstruct deformities and to close defects related to the burn trauma.

Principally, they are:
- Excision techniques
- Serial excision and tissue expansion
- Skin grafting techniques with or without the use of dermal substitutes
- Local skin flaps
- Distant flaps
- Allotransplantation
- Tissue engineering
- Robotics and prosthesis

Fig. 11.2 W-Plasty (*left*) and geometric broken line closure (*right*); (scar: *pink*)

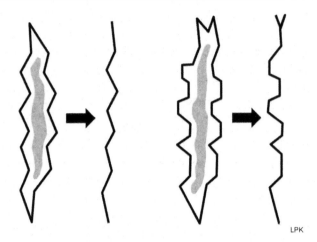

LPK

11.4.1 Excision Techniques

Excision with direct closure of the resultant wound is the simplest and the most direct approach in burn reconstruction. It is important to determine the amount of scar tissue that can be removed so that the resultant defect can be closed directly. A circumferential incision is made in the line previously marked and is carried through the full thickness of the scar down to the subcutaneous fatty layer. In case of a keloid, an intralesional excision might be better instead of an extralesional one in order to avoid recurrence. In order to minimize vascular supply, interference along the wound edges, undermining of the scar edge, should be kept to a minimum, whenever possible.

11.4.1.1 W-Plasty and Geometric Broken Line Closure

The *W-plasty* [8, 9] is a series of connected, triangular advancement flaps mirrored along the length of each side of the scar, but W-plasty, unlike a Z-plasty, does not result in an overall change in length of the scar; it makes the scar less conspicuous, and it disrupts wound contracture with its irregular pattern. As with all other procedures, it is helpful to mark out the planned design prior to the operation (Fig. 11.2).

The geometric broken line closure (GBLC) is a more sophisticated scar regularization technique than the W-plasty and requires more time to execute [10–13]; unlike the W-plasty's regularly irregular pattern, which results in a somewhat predictable scar pattern that can be followed by the observers´ eye, the irregular irregularity of the GBLC allows maximum scar camouflage. This is achieved by various combinations of triangles, rectangles, squares, and semicircles in differing widths and lengths along the scar (Figs. 11.2 and 11.3).

11.4.2 Serial Excision and Tissue Expansion

The goal of surgical reconstruction is the restoration of preoperative function and appearance. The surgeon must reconstruct the defect with tissue of similar contour,

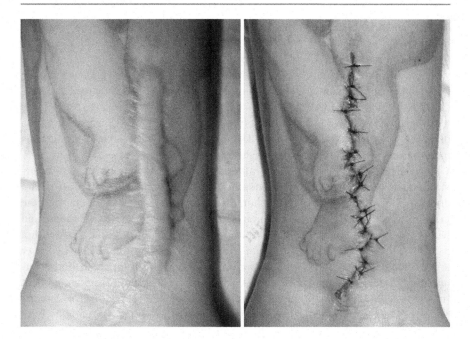

Fig. 11.3 Geometric broken line closure: clinical example

texture, and color. Surgical excision of scars relies upon recruitment of local tissue for closure of the ensuring defect, and thus adjacent skin will usually provide the best match for the defect. In areas where tissue laxity is poor or the resulting defect would be too big, tissue expansion and serial excision are useful techniques to overcome a lack of sufficient local tissue for closure. Tissue expansion allows large areas of burn scar to be resurfaced by providing tissue of similar texture and color to the defect. Moreover, it is combined with the advantage of donor-site morbidity reduction. Issues and disadvantages that need to be addressed are that the technique of pre-expansion requires additional office visits for serial expansion and at least one extra surgical procedure with potential for additional complications. A significant time period between 9 and 12 weeks for progressive tissue expansion is required. Tissue expanders are very versatile tools in reconstructive burn surgery, but still, careful patient selection, correct indications and realistic treatment concepts, large experience and well- selected surgical techniques, precise instruction of the medical staff, as well as detailed and continuous education of the patients are essential [14, 15].

Serial excisions involve the partial excision of the scar with the consecutive advancement of adjunct skin. In a series of sequential procedures, the area of scar is excised completely. The number of procedures needed depends on the elasticity of the surrounding skin and the size of scar being excised. The primary disadvantage of this technique is the requirement for multiple operations. Should more than two operations be needed, tissue expansion should be considered or evaluated as an alternative treatment option.

11.4.3 Skin Grafting Techniques

A Skin Graft without the Combination of a Dermal Substitute – Covering an open wound with a skin graft harvested at a various thickness is the conventional approach of wound closure. A skin graft including epidermis and dermis is defined as a full-thickness skin graft, and a piece of skin cut at a thickness varying between 8/1,000 of an inch (0.196 mm) and 18/1,000 of an inch (0.441 mm) is considered to be a partial- or a split-thickness skin graft. The thickness of a full-thickness skin graft is quite variable depending upon the harvest region.

In case of a full-thickness skin graft, a paper template may be made to determine the size of the skin graft needed to close a wound. The skin graft is laid down to the wound bed and is anchored into place by suturing or stapling the graft onto the wound bed. A continuous contact of the skin graft with the wound bed is essential to ensure an ingrowth of a vascular network in the graft within 3–5 days and thereby for the graft survival. A gauze or cotton bolster tied over a graft has been the traditional technique to anchor and to prevent fluid accumulating underneath a graft, if there is a flat and well-vascularized wound bed. In regions, which are associated with a less good take rate (concave defects; regions, which are subject to repeated motion like joints), or in patients with comorbidities, which may have an impact on graft healing, other techniques [16–18] instead of the bolstering technique are used for skin graft fixation. The use of topical negative pressure or fibrin glue can lead to better skin graft healing [16].

The criteria for using skin grafts of various thicknesses are mainly based on:

- The use of a thin graft is more appropriate for closing wounds with unstable vascular supplies, particularly if the skin graft donor site is scarce.
- Moreover, the quality and the presence of dermis seem to have an influence to the extent of wound contraction. The extent of contraction, which is noted if a thin partial-thickness skin graft is used, is larger than using a full-thickness graft. The presence of a sufficient dermal structure could reduce wound contracture.

Skin Graft in Combination with a Dermal Substitute – For the past several years, artificial dermal substitutes have been used in order to improve skin quality, for example, AlloDerm™ and Integra™ [19]; these materials when implanted over an open wound have been found to form a layer of resembled dermis, thus providing a wound bed better for skin grafting and thereby better skin quality. However, the need for a staged approach to graft a wound using this technique is considered cumbrous. Matriderm ™ is a new dermal matrix, which consists of collagen and elastin and allows a single-step reconstruction of the dermis and epidermis in combination with a split-thickness skin graft [20–22] (Fig. 11.4).

11.4.4 Local Skin Flaps

The approach using a segment of skin with its intrinsic structural components attached to cover a defect follows also the fundamental principle of reconstructive surgery to restore a destructed bodily part with a piece of like tissue. The recent

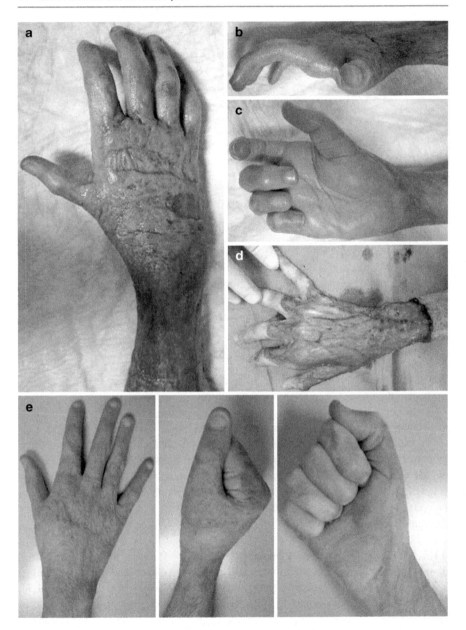

Fig. 11.4 (a) Hypertrophic and contracted scars (*right hand*). (b) Hyperextension in the MCP joints. (c) Flexion only possible in the PIP und DIP joints, hyperextension in the MCP joints. (d) Complete excision of the hypertrophic and contracted scar plate. (e) Late results obtained by use of Matriderm® and skin graft in a single-step procedure (6 months postoperative)

technical innovation of incorporating a muscle and/or facial layer in the skin flap design, especially in a burned area, further expanded the scope of burn reconstruction as more burned tissues could be used for flap fabrication.

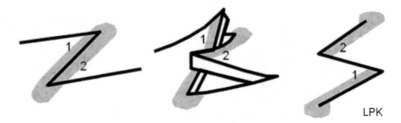

Fig. 11.5 Z-Plasty (scar: *pink*)

No single flap is optimal for every scar excision. Each individual scarred area has to be analyzed for:

- Depth of the scar
- Tissue involved
- Availability of normal tissue for reconstruction

Based on this, the ideal flap or the combination of flaps and techniques is chosen for reconstruction.

Often used skin flaps are the Z-plasty technique, the multiple Z-plasties, and the 3/4 Z-plasty technique.

11.4.4.1 Z-Plasty

There are three purposes to perform a Z-plasty:

- To lengthen a scar or to release a contracture
- To disperse a scar
- To realign a scar within a relaxed skin tension line

The traditional Z-plasty consists of two constant features; first, there are three incisions of equal length – two limbs and a central incision. Second, there are two angles of equal degree – the limbs form 60° angles with the central incision (Fig. 11.6). Ideally, the central incision should go through the axis of the scar; alternatively, the scar itself may be completely excised with a fusiform defect acting as the central incision (Fig. 11.5).

11.4.4.2 Double Opposing Z-Plasty

Two Z-plasty incisions placed immediately adjacent to one another as mirror images will produce an incision known as a double opposing Z-plasty (Figs. 11.6 and 11.7). The advantage of this technique is that significant lengthening can be achieved in areas of limited skin availability. Ideal indication for this technique is the release of web space contractures (Fig. 11.8).

11.4.4.3 ¾ Z-plasty or half-Z

The *¾ Z-plasty or half-Z* is used to refer the technique (Fig. 11.9) with one limb incision being perpendicular to the central one. The incision is created on the scar side, which creates a fissure into the scar in which a triangular flap is introduced. The length gained on the scar side is directly proportional to the width of the triangular flap.

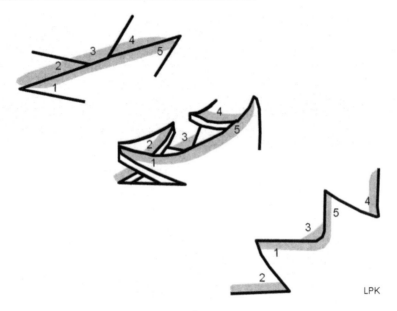

Fig. 11.6 Double opposing Z-plasty (scar: *pink*)

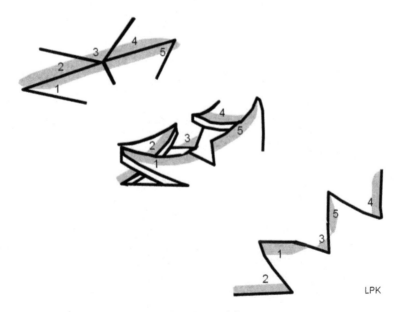

Fig. 11.7 Modified double opposing Z-plasty (scar: *pink*)

Despite its geometric advantage in flap design, fabricating a skin flap or skin flaps for reconstruction of burn deformities is not infrequently plagued with skin necrosis. Aberrant vascular supplies to the skin attributable to the original injury and/or surgical treatment could be the factor responsible for problems. In recent

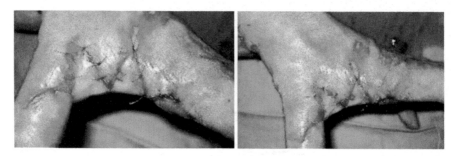

Fig. 11.8 Scar correction by use of a modified double opposing Z-plasty (1 web space)

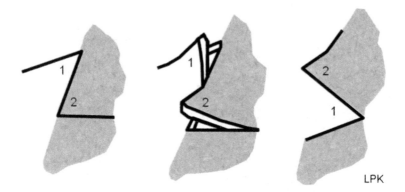

Fig. 11.9 ¾ Z-plasty or half-Z (scar: *pink*)

years, the use of a skin flap designed to include muscle or fascia underneath has expanded further the usefulness of conventional Z-plasty and the 3/4 Z-plasty technique in burn reconstruction.

11.4.4.4 Musculocutaneous (MC) or Fasciocutaneous (FC) Flap Technique

Inclusion of not only the skin but also the subcutaneous tissues and the fascia and the muscle is necessary to fabricate a skin flap to reconstruct a tissue defect in individuals with deep burn injuries. That is, fabricating a flap in a burned area is possible if the underlying muscle or the fascia is included in the design [23].

Moreover, multiple Z-plasties are often used for scar corrections (Figs. 11.10 and 11.11).

11.4.5 Distant Flaps

A distant flap involves a donor site, which is distant from the defect. The mode of transfer might be direct or microvascular. Direct flap, such as the forehead flap or the groin flap, involves direct approximation of the recipient bed to the donor site. These flaps all require a second operation to divide the pedicle.

Fig. 11.10 Multiple
Z-plasties (scar: *pink*)

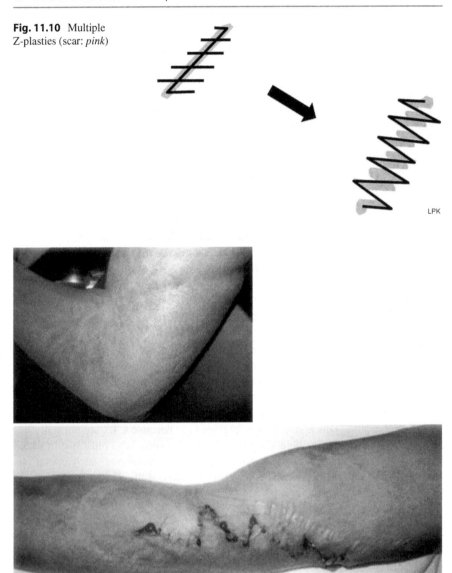

Fig. 11.11 Scar corrections by use of multiple Z-plasties (elbow)

11.4.5.1 Free Tissue Transfer

The evolution of microsurgery and free tissue transfer has dramatically expanded the functional and aesthetic potential of reconstructive surgery. Due to microvascular anastomoses, free transfer of single or compound tissues and replantation of amputated parts are possible. Moreover, by using a free tissue transfer, single-step reconstructions are principally possible.

11.4.5.2 Perforator Flaps

Based on the septocutaneous perforator vessels, the perforator flap was developed. Thus, Song and coworkers described in 1984 [24] that the lateral femur region can serve not only as a skin harvest place but also as the donor site for the "anterolateral thigh (ALT) flap" based on a long pedicle. Then Koshima and colleagues from Japan refined exemplarily the ALT transfer subsequently. In 1989, Koshima introduced an abdominal skin and fat flap based on the inferior epigastric vessels and muscle perforators. Recently, the theory of the perforasomes is under evaluation: Every perforator contains a unique vasculatory territory, the perforasome [25]. This knowledge will lead to new useable pedicled and free flaps for reconstruction.

With the advent of microsurgical techniques, transplanting a composite tissue can be carried out with minimal morbidities. The regimen, in caring for burn victims, however, may be limited because of a paucity of donor materials. It is ironic that burn patients with suitable donor sites seldom require such an elaborate treatment, but those who are in need of microsurgical tissue transplantation are inevitably without appropriate donor sites because of extensive tissue destruction.

11.4.6 Composite Tissue Allotransplantation

"Composite tissue allotransplantation" (CTA) of parts of the face or forearms and upper extremities [26–29] is a young area of transplantation medicine. The first clinical results are promising in comparison to the first reports of the organ transplantation, although the medium-term and long-term problems, for example, tumor induction by the immunosuppression as well as the chronic rejection, have to be taken into account. This is not an unimportant fact, because CTA are normally not of vital importance. Nevertheless, for the affected persons, who must live in social isolation with exhausted reconstructive measures or prostheses, such operations may result a dramatic improvement concerning quality of life. However, it is important to mention that currently only a high selected small number of high motivated patients are candidates for a CTA.

11.4.7 Regeneration: Tissue Engineering

Tissue regeneration and tissue engineering has gained relevance for reconstructive surgery [30–32]. Recently, fat transplantation or lipo transfer is utmost interest. Czerny transplanted in 1895 a lipoma for mamma reconstruction, and fat injection was described among other things by Eugene Holländer in 1910 within a patient with "progressive decrease of the fatty tissue." Erich Lexer dedicated in the first part of his book free fat transfers nearly 300 pages. In 2001, it was demonstrated that beside fat cells also, "adipose-derived stem cells" (ADSC) beside other cell populations in the fatty tissue are usable for these purposes. The transplantation of ADSC was able to regenerate full-layered cartilage defects in the animal model [33]. The stem cell-associated fat cell transplantation in patients with a radioderma has led to improved healing. Moreover, fat cell transplantation is not only able to improve volume and contour defects but also skin quality [34–36]; thereby, it seems that fat transfer will play an important part in burn reconstruction in the future.

11.4.8 Robotics/Prosthesis

If all reconstructive measures fail, myoelectric prostheses are a promising resort to go to. In recent years, these have been improved tremendously by introducing targeted muscle transfers (TMR) to the armamentarium of reconstructive surgery [37, 38]. Modern myoelectric prostheses have multiple degrees of freedom that mandate a complex control system to provide dependable use for the patient. Extremity reconstruction in the twenty-first century will see many new avenues to replace the loss of a limb and reconstruct the loss of function. Both biological and technical advances will provide possibilities that may well open up therapies that have been unthinkable only a few years ago. Targeted muscle reinnervation together with the provision of a myoelectric prosthesis with several degrees of freedom is such an approach and will definitely be a solid stepping stone leading to new strategies in extremity rehabilitation and reconstruction.

11.5 Summary

The regimen of burn treatment has changed drastically over the past 50 years. The regimen of an early debridement and wound coverage, initially with biological dressing and later with autologous skin grafts, had enhanced the survival rate. It is, however, ironic that this improvement in survival rate has caused an increase of patients, who will require reconstructive surgery.

Unsightly hypertrophic scar; scar contracture, affecting particularly the joint structures; and missing bodily parts are still the most common sequelae of burn injuries today.

The difficulty concerning burn reconstruction is largely due to a lack of adequate donor sites, but due to the improvements in reconstructive surgery, better results are achievable. New areas like "composite tissue allotransplantation" of compound tissues like arms or parts of the face, the prosthesis, and also the regenerative medicine with "tissue engineering" have already entered the clinical routine and will improve the final results obtained by burn reconstruction.

References

1. Williams FN, Herndon DN, Hawkins HK et al (2009) The leading causes of death after burn injury in a single pediatric burn center. Crit Care 13(6):183
2. Kamolz LP (2010) Burns: learning from the past in order to be fit for the future. Crit Care 14(1):106
3. Clark JM, Wang TD (2001) Local flaps in scar revision. Facial Plast Surg 4:295–308

4. Mathes S, Nahai F (1982) Clinical application for muscle and musculocutaneous flaps. Mosby, St. Louis
5. Gottlieb LJ, Krieger LM (1994) From the reconstructive ladder to the reconstructive elevator. Plast Reconstr Surg 93(7):1503–1504
6. Knobloch K, Vogt PM (2010) The reconstructive sequence of the 21st century – the reconstructive clockwork. Chirurg 81:441–446
7. Titscher A, Lumenta DB, Kamolz LP et al (2010) Emotional associations with skin: differences between burned and non-burned individuals. Burns 36(6):759–763
8. Borges AF (1959) Improvement of antitension line scar by the "W-plastic" operation. Br J Plast Surg 6:12–29
9. McCarthy JG (1990) Introduction to plastic surgery. In: Plastic surgery. WB Saunders, Philadelphia, pp 1–68
10. Webster RD, Davidson TM, Smith RC (1977) Broken line scar revision. Clin Plast Surg 4:263–274
11. Tardy ME, Thomas RJ, Pashow MS (1981) The camouflage of cutaneous scars. Ear Nose Throat J 60:61–70
12. Alsarraf R, Murakami CS (1998) Geometric broken line closure. Facial Plast Surg Clin North Am 6:163–166
13. Thomas JR (1989) Geometric broken-line closure. In: Thomas JR, Holt GR (eds) Facial scars: incision, revision and camouflage. CV Mosby, St. Louis, pp 160–167
14. Pallua N, von Heimburg D (2005) Pre-expanded ultra-thin supraclavicular flaps for (full-) face reconstruction with reduced donor-site morbidity and without the need for microsurgery. Plast Reconstr Surg 115(7):1837–1844
15. Bozkurt A, Groger A, O'Dey D et al (2008) Retrospective analysis of tissue expansion in reconstructive burn surgery: evaluation of complication rates. Burns 34(8):1113–1118
16. Mittermayr R, Wassermann E, Thurnher M et al (2006) Skin graft fixation by slow clotting fibrin sealant applied as a thin layer. Burns 32(3):305–311
17. Pallua N, Wolter T, Markowicz M (2010) Platelet-rich plasma in burns. Burns 36(1):4–8
18. Roka J, Karle B, Andel H et al (2007) Use of V.A.C. therapy in the surgical treatment of severe burns: the Viennese concept. Handchir Mikrochir Plast Chir 39(5):322–327
19. Nguyen DQ, Potokar TS, Price P (2010) An objective long-term evaluation of Integra (a dermal skin substitute) and split thickness skin grafts, in acute burns and reconstructive surgery. Burns 36(1):23–28
20. Haslik W, Kamolz LP, Nathschläger G et al (2007) First experiences with the collagen-elastin matrix Matriderm as a dermal substitute in severe burn injuries of the hand. Burns 33(3):364–368
21. Haslik W, Kamolz LP, Manna F et al (2010) Management of full-thickness skin defects in the hand and wrist region: first long-term experiences with the dermal matrix Matriderm. J Plast Reconstr Aesthet Surg 63(2):360–364
22. Bloemen MC, van Leeuwen MC, van Vucht NE et al (2010) Dermal substitution in acute burns and reconstructive surgery: a 12-year follow-up. Plast Reconstr Surg 125(5):1450–1459
23. Huang T, Larson DL, Lewis SR (1975) Burned hands. Plast Reconstr Surg 56:21–28
24. Song YG, Chen GZ, Song YL (1984) The free thigh flap: a new free flap concept based on the septocutaneous artery. Br J Plast Surg 37(2):149–159
25. Saint-Cyr M, Wong C, Schaverien M, Mojallal A, Rohrich RJ (2009) The perforasome theory: vascular anatomy and clinical implications. Plast Reconstr Surg 124(5):1529–1544
26. Brandacher G, Ninkovic M, Piza-Katzer H et al (2009) The Innsbruck hand transplant program: update at 8 years after the first transplant. Transplant Proc 41(2):491–494
27. Siemionow MZ, Zor F, Gordon CR (2010) Face, upper extremity, and concomitant transplantation: potential concerns and challenges ahead. Plast Reconstr Surg 126(1):308–315
28. Gordon CR, Siemionow M, Zins J (2009) Composite tissue allotransplantation: a proposed classification system based on relative complexity. Transplant Proc 41(2):481–484
29. Siemionow M, Gordon CR (2010) Overview of guidelines for establishing a face transplant program: a work in progress. Am J Transplant 10(5):1290–1296

30. Kamolz LP, Lumenta DB, Kitzinger HB, Frey M (2008) Tissue engineering for cutaneous wounds: an overview of current standards and possibilities. Eur Surg 40(1):19–26

31. Beier JP, Boos AM, Kamolz L et al (2010) Skin tissue engineering – from split skin to engineered skin grafts? Handchir Mikrochir Plast Chir 42(6):342–353

32. Mansbridge JN (2009) Tissue-engineered skin substitutes in regenerative medicine. Curr Opin Biotechnol 20(5):563–567

33. Dragoo JL, Carlson G, McCormick F et al (2007) Healing full-thickness cartilage defects using adipose-derived stem cells. Tissue Eng 13(7):1615–1621

34. Klinger M, Marazzi M, Vigo D, Torre M (2008) Fat injection for cases of severe burn outcomes: a new perspective of scar remodeling and reduction. Aesthetic Plast Surg 32(3): 465–469

35. Mojallal A, Lequeux C, Shipkov C et al (2009) Improvement of skin quality after fat grafting: clinical observation and an animal study. Plast Reconstr Surg 124(3):765–774

36. Rennekampff HO, Reimers K, Gabka CJ et al (2010) Current perspective and limitations of autologous fat transplantation–"consensus meeting" of the German Society of Plastic, Reconstructive and Aesthetic Surgeons. Handchir Mikrochir Plast Chir 42(2):137–142

37. Aszmann OC, Dietl H, Frey M (2008) Selective nerve transfers to improve the control of myoelectrical arm prostheses. Handchir Mikrochir Plast Chir 40(1):60–65

38. Hijjawi JB, Kuiken TA, Lipschutz RD, Miller LA, Stubblefield KA, Dumanian GA (2006) Improved myoelectric prosthesis control accomplished using multiple nerve transfers. Plast Reconstr Surg 118:1573–1577

Appendix

Sedatives and Pain Medications

Non-intubated patients	Intubated patients
Non-opioid analgesics	Non-opioid analgesics
Acetaminophen (500–1,000 mg po q6h)	Acetaminophen (500–1,000 mg po q6h)
NSAID (Ibuprofen, Naprosyn, Celebrex)	NSAID (Ibuprofen, Naprosyn, Celebrex)
Gabapentin (100–300 mg po q8h) or Pregabalin (50–150 mg po q8h)	Gabapentin (100–300 mg po q8h) or Pregabalin (50–150 mg po q8h)
Opioid analgesics	Opioid analgesics
Morphine (5–20 mg po q4h prn)	IV infusion or prn depending pt requirements
Hydromorphone (1–4 mg po q4h prn)	Morphine (–15 mg IV q1h prn)
	Hydromorphone (0.2–1 mg IV q1–2h prn)
Add long acting opioid analgesics (introduced once 24 h requirements are determined and exceed 30 mg/24 h of morphine or 9 mg/24 h of hydromorphone)	*Add long acting opioid analgesics* (once IV infusion has been discontinued and 24 h oral requirements are determined and exceed 30 mg/24 h of morphine or 9 mg/24 h of hydromorphone)
MS-Contin 10–30 mg po bid/tid	MS-Contin 10–30 mg po bid/tid
Hydromorphone Contin 3–9 mg bid/tid	Hydromorphone Contin 3–9 mg bid/tid
Consider adjuncts specially in those with history of illicit drug abuse and those not responsive to opioids	*Consider adjuncts* specially in those with history of illicit drug abuse and those not responsive to opioids
Ketamine (10–20 mg po tid)	Ketamine (10–20 mg po tid)
Clonidine (0.1–0.2 mg po tid)	Clonidine (0.1–0.2 mg po tid)
Nabilone (1–2 mg po bid)	Nabilone (1–2 mg po bid)

Procedural analgesia/sedation

    Consider Fentanyl IV(up to 1,000 mcg) + Midazolam IV (1–2 mg) for conscious sedation

Or

    Fentanyl (up to 1,000 mcg) IV + Ketamine IV (0.5–2 mg/kg) or Propofol IV (0.5 mg/kg bolus ± 10–20 mg IV incremental boluses) for deep sedation

M.G. Jeschke et al. (eds.), *Burn Care and Treatment*, DOI 10.1007/978-3-7091-1133-8, © Springer-Verlag Wien 2013

Index

M.G. Jeschke et al. (eds.), *Burn Care and Treatment*,
DOI 10.1007/978-3-7091-1133-8, © Springer-Verlag Wien 2013

9 783709 111321